Research Progress on Environmental, Health, and Safety Aspects of **ENGINEERED NANOMATERIALS**

Committee to Develop a Research Strategy for Environmental, Health, and Safety Aspects of Engineered Nanomaterials

Board on Environmental Studies and Toxicology

Board on Chemical Sciences and Technology

National Materials and Manufacturing Board

Division on Earth and Life Studies

Division on Engineering and Physical Sciences

NATIONAL RESEARCH COUNCIL
OF THE NATIONAL ACADEMIES

THE NATIONAL ACADEMIES PRESS
Washington, D.C.
www.nap.edu

THE NATIONAL ACADEMIES PRESS   500 Fifth Street, NW   Washington, DC 20001

NOTICE: The project that is the subject of this report was approved by the Governing Board of the National Research Council, whose members are drawn from the councils of the National Academy of Sciences, the National Academy of Engineering, and the Institute of Medicine. The members of the committee responsible for the report were chosen for their special competences and with regard for appropriate balance.

This project was supported by Contract EP-C-09-003 between the National Academy of Sciences and the US Environmental Protection Agency. Any opinions, findings, conclusions, or recommendations expressed in this publication are those of the authors and do not necessarily reflect the view of the organizations or agencies that provided support for this project.

International Standard Book Number-13: 978-0-309-29186-6
International Standard Book Number-10: 0-309-29186-0

Additional copies of this report are available for sale from the National Academies Press, 500 Fifth Street, NW, Keck 360, Washington, DC 20001; (800) 624-6242 or (202) 334-3313; http://www.nap.edu/.

Copyright 2013 by the National Academy of Sciences. All rights reserved.

Printed in the United States of America

THE NATIONAL ACADEMIES
Advisers to the Nation on Science, Engineering, and Medicine

The **National Academy of Sciences** is a private, nonprofit, self-perpetuating society of distinguished scholars engaged in scientific and engineering research, dedicated to the furtherance of science and technology and to their use for the general welfare. Upon the authority of the charter granted to it by the Congress in 1863, the Academy has a mandate that requires it to advise the federal government on scientific and technical matters. Dr. Ralph J. Cicerone is president of the National Academy of Sciences.

The **National Academy of Engineering** was established in 1964, under the charter of the National Academy of Sciences, as a parallel organization of outstanding engineers. It is autonomous in its administration and in the selection of its members, sharing with the National Academy of Sciences the responsibility for advising the federal government. The National Academy of Engineering also sponsors engineering programs aimed at meeting national needs, encourages education and research, and recognizes the superior achievements of engineers. Dr. C. D. Mote, Jr., is president of the National Academy of Engineering.

The **Institute of Medicine** was established in 1970 by the National Academy of Sciences to secure the services of eminent members of appropriate professions in the examination of policy matters pertaining to the health of the public. The Institute acts under the responsibility given to the National Academy of Sciences by its congressional charter to be an adviser to the federal government and, upon its own initiative, to identify issues of medical care, research, and education. Dr. Harvey V. Fineberg is president of the Institute of Medicine.

The **National Research Council** was organized by the National Academy of Sciences in 1916 to associate the broad community of science and technology with the Academy's purposes of furthering knowledge and advising the federal government. Functioning in accordance with general policies determined by the Academy, the Council has become the principal operating agency of both the National Academy of Sciences and the National Academy of Engineering in providing services to the government, the public, and the scientific and engineering communities. The Council is administered jointly by both Academies and the Institute of Medicine. Dr. Ralph J. Cicerone and Dr. C. D. Mote, Jr., are chair and vice chair, respectively, of the National Research Council.

www.national-academies.org

COMMITTEE TO DEVELOP A RESEARCH STRATEGY FOR ENVIRONMENTAL, HEALTH, AND SAFETY ASPECTS OF ENGINEERED NANOMATERIALS

Members

JONATHAN M. SAMET (*Chair*), University of Southern California, Los Angeles
JURRON BRADLEY, BASF, Florham Park, NJ
SETH COE-SULLIVAN, QD Vision, Inc., Lexington, MA
VICKI L. COLVIN, Rice University, Houston, TX
EDWARD D. CRANDALL, University of Southern California, Los Angeles
RICHARD A. DENISON, Environmental Defense Fund, Washington, DC
WILLIAM H. FARLAND, Colorado State University, Fort Collins
MARTIN FRITTS, SAIC-Frederick, Frederick, MD
PHILIP K. HOPKE, Clarkson University, Potsdam, NY
JAMES E. HUTCHISON, University of Oregon, Eugene
REBECCA D. KLAPER, University of Wisconsin, Milwaukee
GREGORY V. LOWRY, Carnegie Mellon University, Pittsburgh, PA
ANDREW MAYNARD, University of Michigan School of Public Health, Ann Arbor
GÜNTER OBERDÖRSTER, University of Rochester School of Medicine and Dentistry, Rochester, NY
KATHLEEN M. REST, Union of Concerned Scientists, Cambridge, MA
MARK J. UTELL, University of Rochester School of Medicine and Dentistry, Rochester, NY
DAVID B. WARHEIT, DuPont Haskell Global Centers for Health and Environmental Sciences, Newark, DE
MARK R. WIESNER, Duke University, Durham, NC

Staff

EILEEN ABT, Project Director
KERI STOEVER, Research Associate
NORMAN GROSSBLATT, Senior Editor
MIRSADA KARALIC-LONCAREVIC, Manager, Technical Information Center
RADIAH ROSE, Manager, Editorial Projects
CRAIG PHILIP, Senior Program Assistant

Sponsor

US ENVIRONMENTAL PROTECTION AGENCY

BOARD ON ENVIRONMENTAL STUDIES AND TOXICOLOGY[1]

Members

ROGENE F. HENDERSON (*Chair*), Lovelace Respiratory Research Institute, Albuquerque, NM
PRAVEEN AMAR, Clean Air Task Force, Boston, MA
RICHARD A. BECKER, American Chemistry Council, Washington, DC
MICHAEL J. BRADLEY, M.J. Bradley & Associates, Concord, MA
JONATHAN Z. CANNON, University of Virginia, Charlottesville
GAIL CHARNLEY, HealthRisk Strategies, Washington, DC
DAVID C. DORMAN, Department of Molecular Biomedical Sciences, Raleigh, NC
CHARLES T. DRISCOLL, JR., Syracuse University, New York
WILLIAM H. FARLAND, Colorado State University, Fort Collins, CO
LYNN R. GOLDMAN, George Washington University, Washington, DC
LINDA E. GREER, Natural Resources Defense Council, Washington, DC
WILLIAM E. HALPERIN, University of Medicine and Dentistry of New Jersey, Newark
STEVEN P. HAMBURG, Environmental Defense Fund, New York, NY
ROBERT A. HIATT, University of California, San Francisco
PHILIP K. HOPKE, Clarkson University, Potsdam, NY
SAMUEL KACEW, University of Ottawa, Ontario
H. SCOTT MATTHEWS, Carnegie Mellon University, Pittsburgh, PA
THOMAS E. MCKONE, University of California, Berkeley
TERRY L. MEDLEY, E.I. du Pont de Nemours & Company, Wilmington, DE
JANA MILFORD, University of Colorado at Boulder, Boulder
MARK A. RATNER, Northwestern University, Evanston, IL
JOAN B. ROSE, Michigan State University, East Lansing, MI
GINA M. SOLOMON, California Environmental Protection Agency, Sacramento, CA
PETER S. THORNE, University of Iowa, Iowa City, IA
DOMINIC M. DI TORO, University of Delaware Newark, DE
JOYCE S. TSUJI, Exponent Environmental Group, Bellevue, WA

Senior Staff

JAMES J. REISA, Director
DAVID J. POLICANSKY, Scholar
RAYMOND A. WASSEL, Senior Program Officer for Environmental Studies
ELLEN K. MANTUS, Senior Program Officer for Risk Analysis
SUSAN N.J. MARTEL, Senior Program Officer for Toxicology
EILEEN N. ABT, Senior Program Officer
MIRSADA KARALIC-LONCAREVIC, Manager, Technical Information Center
RADIAH ROSE, Manager, Editorial Projects

---

[1]This study was planned, overseen, and supported by the Board on Environmental Studies and Toxicology.

OTHER REPORTS OF THE
BOARD ON ENVIRONMENTAL STUDIES AND TOXICOLOGY

Assessing Risks to Endangered and Threatened Species from Pesticides (2013)
Science for Environmental Protection: The Road Ahead (2012)
Exposure Science in the 21st Century: A Vision and A Strategy (2012)
A Research Strategy for Environmental, Health, and Safety Aspects of Engineered Nanomaterials (2012)
Macondo Well–Deepwater Horizon Blowout: Lessons for Improving Offshore Drilling Safety (2012)
Feasibility of Using Mycoherbicides for Controlling Illicit Drug Crops (2011)
Improving Health in the United States: The Role of Health Impact Assessment (2011)
A Risk-Characterization Framework for Decision-Making at the Food and Drug Administration (2011)
Review of the Environmental Protection Agency's Draft IRIS Assessment of Formaldehyde (2011)
Toxicity-Pathway-Based Risk Assessment: Preparing for Paradigm Change (2010)
The Use of Title 42 Authority at the U.S. Environmental Protection Agency (2010)
Review of the Environmental Protection Agency's Draft IRIS Assessment of Tetrachloroethylene (2010)
Hidden Costs of Energy: Unpriced Consequences of Energy Production and Use (2009)
Contaminated Water Supplies at Camp Lejeune—Assessing Potential Health Effects (2009)
Review of the Federal Strategy for Nanotechnology-Related Environmental, Health, and Safety Research (2009)
Science and Decisions: Advancing Risk Assessment (2009)
Phthalates and Cumulative Risk Assessment: The Tasks Ahead (2008)
Estimating Mortality Risk Reduction and Economic Benefits from Controlling Ozone Air Pollution (2008)
Respiratory Diseases Research at NIOSH (2008)
Evaluating Research Efficiency in the U.S. Environmental Protection Agency (2008)
Hydrology, Ecology, and Fishes of the Klamath River Basin (2008)
Applications of Toxicogenomic Technologies to Predictive Toxicology and Risk Assessment (2007)
Models in Environmental Regulatory Decision Making (2007)
Toxicity Testing in the Twenty-first Century: A Vision and a Strategy (2007)
Sediment Dredging at Superfund Megasites: Assessing the Effectiveness (2007)
Environmental Impacts of Wind-Energy Projects (2007)
Scientific Review of the Proposed Risk Assessment Bulletin from the Office of Management and Budget (2007)
Assessing the Human Health Risks of Trichloroethylene: Key Scientific Issues (2006)
New Source Review for Stationary Sources of Air Pollution (2006)
Human Biomonitoring for Environmental Chemicals (2006)

Health Risks from Dioxin and Related Compounds: Evaluation of the EPA Reassessment (2006)
Fluoride in Drinking Water: A Scientific Review of EPA's Standards (2006)
State and Federal Standards for Mobile-Source Emissions (2006)
Superfund and Mining Megasites—Lessons from the Coeur d'Alene River Basin (2005)
Health Implications of Perchlorate Ingestion (2005)
Air Quality Management in the United States (2004)
Endangered and Threatened Species of the Platte River (2004)
Atlantic Salmon in Maine (2004)
Endangered and Threatened Fishes in the Klamath River Basin (2004)
Cumulative Environmental Effects of Alaska North Slope Oil and Gas Development (2003)
Estimating the Public Health Benefits of Proposed Air Pollution Regulations (2002)
Biosolids Applied to Land: Advancing Standards and Practices (2002)
The Airliner Cabin Environment and Health of Passengers and Crew (2002)
Arsenic in Drinking Water: 2001 Update (2001)
Evaluating Vehicle Emissions Inspection and Maintenance Programs (2001)
Compensating for Wetland Losses Under the Clean Water Act (2001)
A Risk-Management Strategy for PCB-Contaminated Sediments (2001)
Acute Exposure Guideline Levels for Selected Airborne Chemicals (12 volumes, 2000-2012)
Toxicological Effects of Methylmercury (2000)
Strengthening Science at the U.S. Environmental Protection Agency (2000)
Scientific Frontiers in Developmental Toxicology and Risk Assessment (2000)
Ecological Indicators for the Nation (2000)
Waste Incineration and Public Health (2000)
Hormonally Active Agents in the Environment (1999)
Research Priorities for Airborne Particulate Matter (four volumes, 1998-2004)
The National Research Council's Committee on Toxicology: The First 50 Years (1997)
Carcinogens and Anticarcinogens in the Human Diet (1996)
Upstream: Salmon and Society in the Pacific Northwest (1996)
Science and the Endangered Species Act (1995)
Wetlands: Characteristics and Boundaries (1995)
Biologic Markers (five volumes, 1989-1995)
Science and Judgment in Risk Assessment (1994)
Pesticides in the Diets of Infants and Children (1993)
Dolphins and the Tuna Industry (1992)
Science and the National Parks (1992)
Human Exposure Assessment for Airborne Pollutants (1991)
Rethinking the Ozone Problem in Urban and Regional Air Pollution (1991)
Decline of the Sea Turtles (1990)

Copies of these reports may be ordered from the National Academies Press
(800) 624-6242 or (202) 334-3313
www.nap.edu

BOARD ON CHEMICAL SCIENCES AND TECHNOLOGY

Members

DAVID WALT (*Co-chair*), NAE, Tufts University, Medford, Massachusetts
TIMOTHY SWAGER (*Co-chair*), NAS, Massachusetts Institute of Technology, Cambridge
DAVID BEM, The Dow Chemical Company, Midland, Michigan
ROBERT G. BERGMAN, NAS, University of California, Berkeley
JOAN BRENNECKE, NAE, University of Notre Dame, Indiana
HENRY E. BRYNDZA, E. I. du Pont de Nemours & Company, Wilmington, Delaware
DAVID W. CHRISTIANSON, University of Pennsylvania, Philadelphia
RICHARD EISENBERG, NAS, University of Rochester, New York
MARY JANE HAGENSON, Chevron Phillips Chemical Company LLC (retired), The Woodlands, Texas
CAROL J. HENRY, The George Washington University, Washington, D.C.
JILL HRUBY, Sandia National Laboratories, Albuquerque, New Mexico
CHARLES E. KOLB, Aerodyne Research, Inc., Billerica, Massachusetts
SANDER G. MILLS, Merck, Sharp, & Dohme Corporation, Kenilworth, New Jersey
DAVID MORSE, NAE, Corning Incorporated, Corning, New York
ROBERT E. ROBERTS, Institute for Defense Analyses, Alexandria, Virginia
DARLENE SOLOMON, Agilent Technologies, Santa Clara, California
JEAN TOM, Bristol-Myers Squibb, West Windsor, New Jersey

Senior Staff

DOROTHY ZOLANDZ, Director
KATHRYN HUGHES, Senior Program Officer
DOUGLAS FRIEDMAN, Program Officer
ELIZABETH FINKELMAN, Administrative Assistant

OTHER REPORTS OF THE BOARD ON CHEMICAL SCIENCES AND TECHNOLOGY

Opportunities and Obstacles in Large-Scale Biomass Utilization: The Role of the Chemical Sciences and Engineering Communities: A Workshop Summary (2013)
Determining Core Capabilities in Chemical and Biological Defense Science and Technology (2012)
Transforming Glycoscience: A Roadmap for the Future (2012)
Assuring a Future U.S.-Based Nuclear and Radiochemistry Expertise (2012)
The Use and Storage of Methyl Isocyanate at Bayer CropScience (2012)
Challenges in Chemistry Graduate Education: A Workshop Summary (2012)
The Role of the Chemical Sciences in Finding Alternatives to Critical Resources: A Workshop Summary (2012)
Challenges in Characterizing Small Particles: Exploring Particles from the Nano- to Microscales: A Workshop Summary (2012)
Research Frontiers in Bioinspired Energy: Molecular-Level Learning from Natural Systems: A Workshop (2012)
Chemistry in Primetime and Online: Communicating Chemistry in Informal Environments (2011)
Prudent Practices in the Laboratory: Handling and Management of Chemical Hazards, Revised Edition (2011)
Trends in Science and Technology Relevant to the Biological and Toxin Weapons Convention: Summary of an International Workshop: October 31 to November 3, 2010, Beijing, China (2011)
Promoting Chemical Laboratory Safety and Security in Developing Countries (2010)
Research at the Intersection of the Physical and Life Sciences (2010)
BioWatch and Public Health Surveillance: Evaluating Systems for the Early Detection of Biological Threats: Abbreviated Version (2010)
Strengthening High School Chemistry Education Through Teacher Outreach Programs: A Workshop Summary to the Chemical Sciences Roundtable (2009)
Catalysis for Energy: Fundamental Science and Long-Term Impacts of the U.S. Department of Energy Basic Energy Science Catalysis Science Program (2009)
Effectiveness of National Biosurveillance Systems: BioWatch and the Public Health System: Interim Report (2009)
A Framework for Assessing the Health Hazard Posed by Bioaerosols (2008)
Disrupting Improvised Explosive Device Terror Campaigns: Basic Research Opportunities: A Workshop Report (2008)
Test and Evaluation of Biological Standoff Detection Systems: Abbreviated Version (2008)

NATIONAL MATERIALS AND MANUFACTURING BOARD

Members

ROBERT E. SCHAFRIK (*Chair*), NAE, General Electric Aviation, Cincinnati, OH
PETER R. BRIDENBAUGH, NAE, Aluminum Company of America (retired), Boca Raton, FL
LAWRENCE D. BURNS, NAE, University of Michigan, Franklin
JIM C. CHANG, National Cheng Kung University, Taiwan
GEORGE (RUSTY) T. GRAY, III, Los Alamos National Laboratory, Los Alamos, NM
JENNIE S. HWANG, NAE, H-Technologies Group, Inc., Cleveland, OH
SUNDARESAN JAYARAMAN, Georgia Institute of Technology, Atlanta
MAJ. GEN ROBERT H. LATIFF, R. Latiff Associates, Alexandria, VA
MICHAEL F. MCGRATH, ANSER (Analytic Services Inc.), Arlington, VA
CELIA MERZBACHER, Semiconductor Research Corporation, Research Triangle Park, NC
EDWARD MORRIS, National Center for Defense Manufacturing and Machining, Youngstown, OH
ROBERT C. PFAHL, JR., International Electronics Manufacturing Initiative, Herndon, VA
VINCENT J. RUSSO, Aerospace Technologies Associates, LLC, Dayton, OH
HAYDN N. WADLEY, University of Virginia, Charlottesville
BEN WANG, Georgia Institute of Technology, Atlanta
ALBERT R. C. WESTWOOD, NAE, Sandia National Laboratories, Albuquerque, NM

Senior Staff

DENNIS CHAMOT, Acting Director
ERIK B. SVEDBERG, Senior Program Officer
HEATHER LOZOWSKI, Financial Manager
JOSEPH PALMER, Senior Program Assistant

OTHER REPORTS OF THE NATIONAL MATERIALS AND MANUFACTURING BOARD

Optics and Photonics: Essential Technologies for our Nation (2012)
Engineering Aviation Security Environments – Reduction of False Alarms in Computed Tomography-Based Screening of Checked Baggage (2012)
Application of Lightweighting Technology to Military Vehicles, Vessels, and Aircraft (2011)
Opportunities in Protection Materials Science and Technology for Future Army Applications (2011)
Materials Needs and R&D Strategy for Future Military Aerospace Propulsion Systems (2011)
Research Opportunities in Corrosion Science and Engineering (2010)
Assessment of Corrosion Education (2009)
Proceedings of a Workshop on Materials State Awareness (2008)
Integrated Computational Materials Engineering: A Transformational Discipline for Improved Competitiveness and National Security (2008)
Managing Materials for a Twenty-first Century Military (2008)
A Path to the Next Generation of U.S. Bank Notes: Keeping Them Real (2007)
Assessment of Millimeter-Wave and Terahertz Technology for Detection and Identification of Concealed Explosives and Weapons (2007)
Fusion of Security System Data to Improve Airport Security (2007)
Proceedings of the Materials Forum 2007: Corrosion Education for the 21st Century (2007)
Managing Materials for a 21st Century Military (2007)
A Matter of Size: Triennial Review of the National Nanotechnology Initiative (2006)
Proceedings from the Workshop on Biomedical Materials at the Edge: Challenges in the Convergence of Technologies (2006)
Defending the U.S. Air Transportation System Against Chemical and Biological Threats (2006)
Globalization of Materials R&D: Time for a National Strategy (2005)
Going to Extremes: Meeting the Emerging Demand for Durable Polymer Matrix Composites (2005)
High-Performance Structural Fibers for Advanced Polymer Matrix Composites (2005)
Nanotechnology for the Intelligence Community (2005)

Preface

Over the last decade, there has been an increase in funding for research on and a rising number of publications that address the environmental, health, and safety (EHS) aspects of engineered nanomaterials (ENMs). Those efforts have led to progress in understanding some aspects of potential EHS risks posed by ENMs. However, research on the potential EHS implications of ENMs still lacks context, particularly with regard to future risks, because uses of materials are changing rapidly. EHS research efforts are not keeping pace with the evolving applications of nanotechnology, and uncertainty persists about the potential implications of the materials for consumers, workers, and ecosystems. To address those uncertainties, the Environmental Protection Agency asked the National Research Council to perform an independent study to develop and monitor the implementation of an integrated research strategy to address the EHS aspects of ENMs. In response to that request, the Committee to Develop a Research Strategy for Environmental, Health, and Safety Aspects of Engineered Nanomaterials was formed and released a report in January 2012, *A Research Strategy for the Environmental, Health, and Safety Aspects of Engineered Nanomaterials.* That report developed a research plan with short-term and long-term priorities and estimated resources needed to implement the research plan.

In this second report, the committee assesses the trajectory of research progress on the basis of indicators identified in its first report. The committee suggests pathways for advancing the research and considers a vision for optimizing the research efforts of the nanotechnology EHS community.

This report has been reviewed in draft form by persons chosen for their diverse perspectives and technical expertise in accordance with procedures approved by the National Research Council Report Review Committee. The purposes of the independent review are to provide candid and critical comments that will assist the institution in making its published report as sound as possible and to ensure that the report meets institutional standards of objectivity, evidence, and responsiveness to the study charge. The review comments and draft manuscript remain confidential to protect the integrity of the deliberative process. We thank the following for their review of this report: Nathan Baker, Pacific Northwest National Laboratory; Diana Bowman, University of Michigan; Barbara Boyan, Virginia Commonwealth University; Elsa Garmire, Dartmouth College; Timothy Killeen, State

University of New York, Albany; Terry Medley, E.I. duPont de Nemours & Co.; Andre Nel, University of California, Los Angeles; Robert Tanguay, Oregon State University; Jason Unrine, University of Kentucky; and Paul Westerhoff, Arizona State University.

Although the reviewers listed above have provided many constructive comments and suggestions, they were not asked to endorse the conclusions or recommendations, nor did they see the final draft of the report before its release. The review of the report was overseen by the review coordinator, Richard B. Schlesinger, Pace University, and the review monitor, Julia M. Phillips, Sandia National Laboratories. Appointed by the National Research Council, they were responsible for making certain that an independent examination of the report was carried out in accordance with institutional procedures and that all review comments were carefully considered. Responsibility for the final content of the report rests entirely with the committee and the institution.

The committee gratefully acknowledges the following for making presentations to the committee during its November 7, 2012 workshop in Washington, DC (see Appendix C for a summary of the workshop): James Alwood and Tina Bahadori, US Environmental Protection Agency; Nathan Baker, Pacific Northwest National Laboratory; Carolyn Cairns, Consumers Union; Teresa Croce, US Food and Drug Administration; Anna Fendley, United Steel Workers; Charles Geraci and Paul Schulte, National Institute for Occupational Safety and Health; Vincent Hackley, National Institute of Standards and Technology; Michael Holman, Lux Research; Barbara Karn, National Science Foundation; Georgios Katalagarianakis, European Commission; Jamie Lead, University of South Carolina; Scott McNeil, National Cancer Institute; Sri Nadadur and Christopher Weis, National Institute of Environmental Health Sciences; Martin Philbert, University of Michigan; Mihail Roco, National Science Foundation; Robert (Skip) Rung, Oregon Nanoscience and Microtechnologies Institute; Maxine Savitz, Honeywell Corporation (retired); Robert Tanguay, Oregon State University; and Sally Tinkle, Science Technology and Policy Institute (formerly with the National Nanotechnology Coordination Office).

The committee is also grateful for the assistance of National Research Council staff in preparing this report: Eileen Abt, project director; James Reisa, director of the Board on Environmental Studies and Toxicology; Keri Stoever, research associate; Norman Grossblatt, senior editor; Mirsada Karalic-Loncarevic, manager, Technical Information Center; Radiah Rose, manager, editorial projects; and Craig Philip, senior program assistant.

I would especially like to thank the members of the committee for their efforts throughout the development of this report.

                              Jonathan M. Samet, *Chair*
                              Committee to Develop a Research
                              Strategy for Environmental, Health, and
                              Safety Aspects of Engineered Nanomaterials

Contents

SUMMARY 3

1   INTRODUCTION 17
      Study Scope, 18
      Overview of First Report, 19
      Context for and Approach to Second Report, 24
      References, 26

2   REVIEW OF RECENT REPORTS AND NATIONAL
      RESEARCH COUNCIL COMMITTEE WORKSHOP 28
      Introduction, 28
      The National Nanotechnology Initiative Supplement to the
         President's FY 2013 Budget, 29
      The Report to the President and Congress on the Fourth
         Assessment of the National Nanotechnology Initiative, 30
      Government Accountability Office Report, Nanotechnology:
         Improved Performance Information Needed for
         Environmental, Health, and Safety Research, 31
      European Union Efforts, 34
      National Research Council Committee Workshop, 37
      Conclusion, 37
      References, 38

3   ASSESSMENT OF PROGRESS 41
      Introduction, 41
      Indicators of Research Progress, 43
      Indicators of Progress in Implementation, 67
      References, 73

4   GETTING TO GREEN 83
      Introduction, 83
      Fundamental Processes Affecting Nanomaterial Exposure
         and Hazard, 86

Nanomaterial Sources and Development of Reference Materials, 87
Model Development, 90
Methods and Instrumentation, 92
Informatics: The Knowledge Commons, 94
Nanomaterial Interactions in Complex Systems Ranging from Subcellular Systems to Ecosystems, 98
Analysis of Progress Towards Addressing Implementation Needs, 101
References, 111

5 GOING BEYOND GREEN 115
Introduction: A Vision for the Future, 115
Effective Governance, 117
Sustaining and Nurturing Research Excellence, 121
Adaptive Decision-Making and Knowledge-Sharing, 122
Conclusion, 125
References, 125

APPENDIXES

A BIOGRAPHIC INFORMATION ON THE COMMITTEE TO DEVELOP A RESEARCH STRATEGY FOR ENVRIONMENTAL, HEALTH, AND SAFETY ASPECTS OF ENGINEERED NANOMATERIALS 126

B STATEMENT OF TASK 135

C WORKSHOP SUMMARY: RESEARCH PROGRESS ON ENVIRONMENTAL, HEALTH, AND SAFETY ASPECTS OF NANOTECHNOLOGY 137

BOXES AND FIGURES

BOXES

S-1 Status of Indicators of Progress in Research, 6
S-2 Status of Indicators of Progress in Implementation, 8
1-1 Research-Progress Indicators, 22
1-2 Indicators of Progress in Implementation, 23
3-1 Status of Indicators of Research Progress, 42
3-2 Status of Indicators of Progress in Implementation, 44

FIGURES

S-1   Nanotechnology environmental, health, and safety
          research enterprise, 5
1-1   Conceptual framework for the committee's research strategy, 20
1-2   Nanotechnology environmental, health, and safety
          research enterprise, 25
4-1   Nanotechnology environmental, health, and safety
          research enterprise, 84

Research Progress on Environmental, Health, and Safety Aspects of **ENGINEERED NANOMATERIALS**

Summary

Nanotechnology relies on the ability to design, manipulate, and manufacture materials at the nanoscale.[1] Investments in nanotechnology and in the production of engineered nanomaterials (ENMs) continue to grow; the global market for nanotechnology is expected to exceed $3 trillion by 2015. The novel physical and chemical characteristics of ENMs are being exploited in new applications and have motivated research on the potential human health and environmental risks associated with these materials because of concerns about their behavior in biologic systems. Given the global use of ENMs, research on their environmental, health, and safety (EHS) aspects necessarily extends globally and involves a multidisciplinary and international group of stakeholders, including academic researchers, the industrial sector, nongovernment organizations (NGOs), and the public.

Over the last decade, there has been more funding for research and a corresponding increase in peer-reviewed publications on EHS aspects of ENMs. However, in spite of progress in understanding some aspects of risks posed by ENMs, uncertainty persists about the potential implications of the materials for consumers, workers, and ecosystems. In that context, the US Environmental Protection Agency (EPA) asked the National Research Council to perform an independent study to develop and monitor an integrated research strategy on EHS risks posed by ENMs.

In response to EPA's request, the National Research Council convened the Committee to Develop a Research Strategy for Environmental, Health, and Safety Aspects of Engineered Nanomaterials, which produced its first report in 2012, *A Research Strategy for Environmental, Health, and Safety Aspects of Engineered Nanomaterials*. In this second report, the committee evaluates the trajectory of research progress on the basis of indicators or criteria established in its first report. (See Appendix B for complete statement of task.) This report expands on the need for a strategic approach for developing the research infrastructure for addressing uncertainties regarding the potential EHS risks associated with ENMs that was begun in the first report. The approach hinges on the vision put forth in Figure S-1, which describes the nanotechnology EHS research enterprise and shows the interrelated and interdependent research activities that are driven by the production of

---

[1] *Nanoscale* refers to materials on the order of one billionth of a meter.

ENMs. The diagram presents an integrated and strategic system for developing data that will provide for characterization of ENMs, for refinement of experimental methods, for support of model development, and for storage and retrieval of information through the "knowledge commons". The potential success of the enterprise rests on involvement of the global community of stakeholders, including researchers, manufacturers of ENMs, regulators, and components of civil society that are invested in addressing potential health and environmental risks posed by ENMs. Many of the elements of this enterprise are in place, but the committee concludes that their further development and integration are essential for advancing progress.

The committee's second report considers findings that were presented in its first report and other recently released US and European Union efforts that provide global perspectives for advancing nanotechnology EHS research. It examines trajectories of research and implementation progress and identifies barriers to progress and steps to ensure progress. To advance the concepts described in the research enterprise (Figure S-1), the committee envisions a time beyond its current research recommendations to consider how questions about risk can be best approached in an adaptive fashion with the goal of generating information needed to design materials and processes so as to avoid and control potential risks.

ASSESSMENT OF PROGRESS

This report is released a short time after of the committee's first report. Using indicators developed based on priorities from that report (see Boxes S-1 and S-2 for indicators of research and implementation progress, respectively), the committee evaluated progress in this second report.

For its evaluation, the committee developed a color scheme to categorize progress qualitatively by considering new activities since preparation of its first report and the trajectory of research progress. Because of the many concomitant nanotechnology EHS reviews and planning efforts, the committee did not attempt to attribute progress to any particular effort. Rather, it classified progress on the basis of committee consensus whereby **green** implies substantial progress (there are new activities, and sustained progress is expected), **yellow** implies moderate or mixed progress, and **red** implies little progress (there is minimal activity, and little change is expected). (The committee's assessment of progress is indicated in the color circles in Boxes S-1 and S-2.)

In the following sections, the committee provides a brief evaluation of the research and implementation indicators, together with the steps needed to speed progress to a pace at which "getting to green"[2] is achievable. (Additional details regarding the evaluation of progress are described in Chapters 3 and 4.)

---

[2]"Getting to green" is the title of Chapter 4, and indicates the steps needed to achieve progress in the research and implementation indicators identified in Boxes S-1 and S-2.

Summary 5

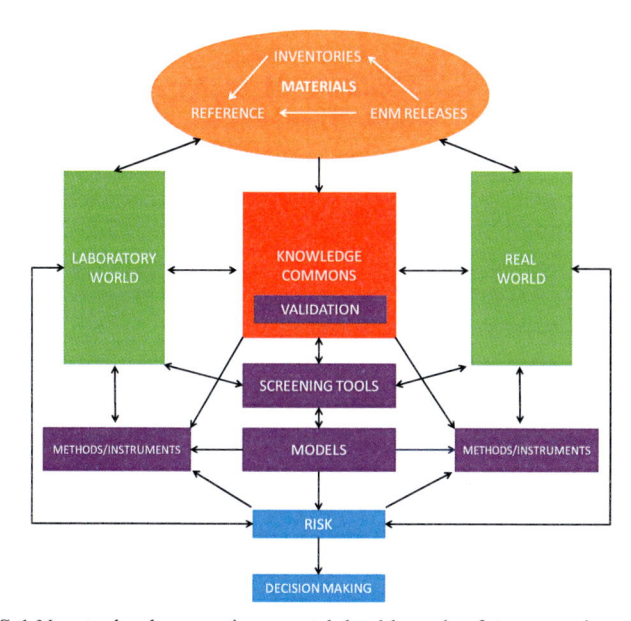

FIGURE S-1 Nanotechnology environmental, health, and safety research enterprise. The diagram shows the integrated and interdependent research activities that are driven by the production of ENMs. The production of ENMs is captured by the orange oval, labeled "materials", which includes reference materials, ENM releases, and inventories. (An inventory is a quantitative estimate of the location and amounts of nanomaterials produced, including the properties of the nanomaterial.) The knowledge commons (red box) is the locus for collaborative development of methods, models, and materials, and for archiving and sharing data. The "laboratory world" and "real world" (green boxes) feed into the knowledge commons. The laboratory world comprises process-based and mechanism-based research that is directed at understanding the physical, chemical, and biologic properties or processes that are most critical for assessing exposures and hazards and hence risk (NRC 2012, p. 55). The "real world" includes complex systems research involving observational studies that examine the effects of ENMs on people and ecosystems. The purple boxes capture the range of methods, tools, models, and instruments that support generation of research in the laboratory world, the real world, and the knowledge commons.

Research Progress

Adaptive Research and Knowledge Infrastructure for Accelerating Research Progress and Providing Rapid Feedback to Advance Research

In the first report, the committee identified a need for an adaptive infrastructure for research and knowledge generation to accelerate and advance nanotechnology EHS research. The components of the infrastructure include characterized materials for reference and research purposes; nanomaterial libraries;

instruments and methods for measuring nanomaterials and their transformations; methods or assays for quantifying the effects of nanomaterials; databases, ontologies[3], and tools for sharing research results; and models for uncovering relationships among the data. In this second report, the committee determined that research progress ranges from green for detecting and characterizing ENMs in relatively well-characterized media to yellow for development of libraries of well-characterized ENMs, development of methods for quantifying effects of ENMs in experimental systems, and the extent of joining existing databases and advancing systems for sharing research results.

BOX S-1 Status of Indicators of Progress in Research[4]

Adaptive Research and Knowledge Infrastructure for Accelerating Research Progress and Providing Rapid Feedback to Advance the Research

- Extent of development of libraries of well-characterized nanomaterials, including those prevalent in commerce and reference and standard materials
- Development of methods for detecting, characterizing, tracking, and monitoring nanomaterials and their transformations in simple, well-characterized media
- Development of methods to quantify effects of nanomaterials in experimental systems.
- Extent of joining of existing databases, including development of common informatics ontologies
- Advancement of systems for sharing the results of research and fostering development of predictive models of nanomaterial behaviors

Quantifying and Characterizing the Origins of Nanomaterial Releases

- Developing inventories of current and near-term production of nanomaterials
- Developing inventories of intended uses of nanomaterials and value-chain transfers
- Identifying critical release points along the value chain
- Identifying critical populations or systems exposed
- Characterizing released materials in complex environments
- Modeling nanomaterial releases along the value chain

(Continued)

---

[3]Ontologies—specifications of the terms and their logical relationships used in a particular field—are used to improve search capabilities and allow mapping of relationships among databases and informatics systems.

[4]The wording and ordering of some indicators have been modified from NRC (2012, pp. 181–182). Details of the modifications are noted in the descriptions of the indicators in Chapter 3.

> **BOX S-1** Continued
>
> **Processes That Affect Both Exposure and Hazard**
>
> - Steps taken toward development of a knowledge infrastructure able to describe the diversity and dynamics of nanomaterials and their transformations in complex biologic and environmental media
> - Progress in developing instrumentation to measure key nanomaterial properties and changes in them in complex biologic and environmental media
> - Initiation of interdisciplinary research that can relate native nanomaterial structures to transformations that occur in organisms and as a result of biologic processes
> - Extent of use of experimental research results in initial models for predicting nanomaterial behavior in complex biologic and environmental settings
>
> **Nanomaterial Interactions in Complex Systems Ranging from Subcellular Systems to Ecosystems**
>
> - Extent of initiation of studies that address the impacts of nanomaterials on a variety of end points in complex systems, such as studies that link in vitro to in vivo observations, that examine effects on important biologic pathways, and that investigate ecosystem effects
> - Extent of adaptation of existing system-level tools (such as individual species tests, microcosms, and organ-system models) to support studies of nanomaterials in such systems
> - Development of a set of screening tools that reflect important characteristics or toxicity pathways of the complex systems described above
> - Steps toward development of models for exposure and potential ecologic effects
> - Identification of benchmark (positive and negative) and reference materials for use in such studies and measurement tools and methods to estimate exposure and dose in complex systems

Quantifying and Characterizing the Origins of Material Releases

Knowledge of human and ecosystem exposures requires detailed information on the quantities and characteristics of ENMs produced and the products in which they are used, on how they are introduced into the environment, on how they are transported and transformed in humans and ecosystems, and on the populations exposed.

Progress in this research priority ranged from yellow to red. Yellow was assigned for the extent of progress in developing inventories of ENMs, in identifying critical release points along the value chain, in identifying critical populations or systems exposed, and in characterizing released materials in complex environments. Because those are prerequisites for model development, the ability to model releases along the value chain was denoted as red.

> **BOX S-2** Status of Indicators of Progress
> in Implementation (NRC 2012, p. 183)
>
> **Enhancing Interagency Coordination**
>
> - Progress toward establishing a mechanism to ensure sufficient management and budgetary authority to develop and implement an EHS-research strategy among NNI agencies
> - Extent to which the NNCO is annually identifying funding needs for interagency collaboration on critical high-priority research
>
> **Providing for Stakeholder Engagement in the Research Strategy**
>
> - Progress toward actively engaging diverse stakeholders in a continuing manner in all aspects of strategy development, implementation, and revision
>
> **Conducting and Communicating the results of research funded through public-private partnerships**
>
> - Progress toward establishment of effective public-private partnerships, as measured by such steps as completion of partnership agreements, issuance of requests for proposal, and establishment of a sound governance structure
>
> **Managing Potential Conflicts of Interest**
>
> - Progress toward achieving a clear separation in management and budgetary authority and accountability between the functions of developing and promoting applications of nanotechnology and understanding and assessing its potential health and environmental implications
> - Continued separate tracking and reporting of EHS research activities and funding distinct from those for other, more basic or application-oriented research

Processes that Affect Both Exposure and Hazard

In its first report, the committee highlighted the need to identify the critical nanomaterial interactions that affect ENM behaviors and recommended identifying cross-cutting processes common to assessing exposure and hazard. This topic includes cataloging the types of ENM transformations in complex matrices, developing instrumentation for monitoring transformations in vivo or in complex environmental media, and developing models for predicting ENM behaviors. There is a need for an infrastructure for archiving data on ENM behavior for model development. Progress ranged from yellow for initiation of studies to characterize ENM transformations and for studies that relate ENM properties to observed effects in more complex systems to red for development of new instrumentation for measuring transformations in situ, in vivo, or in single particles.

Nanomaterial Interactions in Complex Systems Ranging from Subcellular Systems to Ecosystems

In its first report, the committee recognized the need to improve understanding of interactions of ENMs in a variety of complex systems—from single cells to subcellular organelles to individual organisms to ecosystems. A first step is to identify relevant exposure sources, concentrations, and cellular, organismal, and ecologic targets so that potential effects on complex systems can be addressed. Research progress indicators for this category ranged from yellow to red with none denoted as green. Indicators were yellow for initiation of studies that address effects of ENMs in complex systems, adaptation of system-level tools to support studies of these systems, and steps toward development of models for assessing ecologic exposures and effects. Indicators were red for developing screening tools that reflect important toxicity pathways and for identifying benchmark and reference ENMs for use in studies to characterize exposure or dose.

Research Progress Indicators: Getting to Green

The research enterprise (Figure S-1) provides a means of capturing the flow of activities and examining the pathways needed to advance research progress to get to green. As such the figure provides a means of illustrating barriers to research progress. The discussion focuses on six major categories: nanomaterial sources and development of reference materials, processes that affect nanomaterial exposure and hazard, the knowledge commons, model development, methods and instrumentation, and nanomaterial interactions in complex systems.

Nanomaterial Sources and Development of Reference Materials

Relevant ENMs include reference materials, materials from inventories, and materials released and modified across their value chain and life cycle. ENMs form the central element of research studies in the knowledge commons, the laboratory world, and the real world. The appropriate design and characterization of ENMs are needed for developing libraries, informing the design of future ENMs, developing the data to populate the knowledge commons, developing new methods and instrumentation, and conducting mechanistic studies and studies in complex media.

The nanotechnology EHS research community has relied on commonly available ENMs to conduct most studies. There is no process for determining which nanomaterials should have high priority for development on the basis of research needs. Elements for advancing the development and distribution of reference nanomaterials for research and analytic purposes to get to green include the following:

- A mechanism for identifying and setting priorities among nanomaterials and libraries for development.
- Adoption and use of appropriate and standardized material descriptors for the design, development, and sharing of ENMs.
- Improved synthesis and purification methods for ENMs.
- Collaboration among the scientists who are studying mechanisms and complex systems to optimize materials for study.
- New methods and approaches for rapid characterization of reference materials.
- Instrumentation for characterizing complex nanoscale species (materials of unknown origin, mixtures, and released materials).
- Information-management plans and appropriate research infrastructure for collecting information on nanomaterial production and uses along the value chain.

Fundamental Processes That Affect Nanomaterial Exposure and Hazard

Research in this category occurs both in the laboratory world and the real world (Figure S-1) and involves experimental approaches to understand the physical, chemical, and biologic processes that affect exposure and hazard. Hypothesized ENM properties are scrutinized in well-defined laboratory experiments and in observations of ENM behavior in complex systems, from in vivo experiments to models of ecosystem interactions. The research is informed by development of methods and instrumentation that are needed for understanding ENM transformations, distribution, and effects.

Continued efforts to elucidate mechanisms of ENM interactions with organisms and ecosystems are critical for achieving the long-term goal of predicting ENM effects. The ability to make such predictions will allow evaluation of risks posed by ENMs at the design stage, in model predictions, and in validated screening assays. Continued progress in understanding mechanisms of ENM behavior will require advances in instrument development and an improved data-integration infrastructure.

Informatics: The Knowledge Commons

The knowledge commons, the focal point of Figure S-1, is the locus for collaborative development of methods, models, and materials, and its success requires increased integration with research in the laboratory world and the real world and with development of materials. The knowledge commons serves three functions: a collaborative environment for the development and validation of predictive models, a collaborative environment for methods development, and a collaborative environment for the design of ENMs with the objective of improving manufacturing processes to reduce risks.

The strength of the knowledge commons is its ability to knit existing and new capabilities together in an overarching framework that provides a means of linking the various components of nanotechnology EHS research; such integration has not yet occurred. In addition, such new initiatives as the National Nanotechnology Initiative (NNI) Nanotechnology Knowledge Infrastructure (NKI) and the Materials Genome Initiative could augment the knowledge commons by providing additional linkages and informatics expertise. The knowledge commons would also have a key role in integrating participation of all sectors—including government and academic researchers, NGOs, regulators, and industry—to generate the data and knowledge that are required as inputs.

Model Development

An important outcome of the knowledge commons will be the development of a suite of models for predicting physical characteristics of ENMs, outcomes of toxicity testing, and exposures. There has been some progress in development of some types of models, but there is a lack of consistency in approaches and interoperability of data to support effective model development. Development of integrated models is needed to link behavior of ENMs to their characteristics and to properties of systems into which they are released.

Getting to green in the development of predictive models will require substantial data development from mechanistic and complex-system studies and characterization of physical properties of a variety of ENMs in different environments. Initial models will need to be developed iteratively using emerging data. Early outputs of the models can inform data needs and influence decisions about experimental approaches and instrumentation needs.

Methods and Instrumentation

Methods and instrumentation are defined as tools required for detecting and characterizing ENMs and their properties in relevant media. Progress in development of methods and instrumentation has varied because of the different applications of the tools; there has been some progress in characterizing newly manufactured ENMs in well-understood, simple media but little in detecting and characterizing ENMs in complex environments.

Progress in developing methods and instrumentation will require characterization and quantification of the properties of ENMs in complex biologic and environmental media and measurement of the properties of single particles so that specific ENM properties can be associated with observed behaviors and effects.

Nanomaterial Interactions in Complex Systems Ranging from Subcellular Systems to Ecosystems

Research on nanomaterial interactions in complex systems cuts across the laboratory world and the real world (Figure S-1). A critical barrier to advancing understanding of ENM interactions in complex systems is the lack of mechanistic data: an increasing volume of toxicity data is being produced, but the ability to use the data to predict ENM risks with any certainty is constrained because of the types of studies conducted. To provide more useful information on potential human and environmental risk, studies need to focus on more complex experimental-design issues—such as relevant dose and dosimetry; dose–response relationships and time-course characteristics; appropriate target cells, tissues, and organisms; and examination of more biologic pathways—concomitantly with better characterization of ENM test substances and incorporation of standardized reference materials as controls.

The data, in a common format, should be shared among investigators, and results of in vivo studies (at relevant concentrations) should be compared with results of in situ and in vitro screening assays to foster development of these more expedient testing strategies. Validated screening tools also need to be developed so that information can be compared across experiments and used in modeling efforts to predict potential effects on humans and ecosystems.

Implementation Progress and Steps Needed to Get to Green

In the committee's first report, it identified mechanisms to ensure implementation of the EHS research strategy: enhancing interagency coordination; providing for stakeholder engagement in the research strategy; conducting and communicating results of research funded through public–private partnerships; and managing conflicts of interest. Collectively, those mechanisms represent support needed for the nanotechnology EHS research enterprise (Figure S-1), given the broad potential reach of nanotechnology in our society and economy and the EHS issues that span the missions of many stakeholders. Progress in addressing implementation indicators ranged from yellow to red; no indicators were denoted as green (see Box S-2).

Enhancing Interagency Coordination

In its first report, the committee acknowledged the value of the coordinating role played by NNI and pointed to changes that have enhanced interagency coordination, including the naming of an EHS coordinator to the National Nanotechnology Coordination Office (NNCO) and the NNI's release of its 2011 EHS research strategy. However, the committee concluded that accountability for implementation of the NNI's EHS research strategy is hampered by the absence of an entity that has sufficient management and budgetary authority to direct

Summary 13

implementation among NNI agencies and to ensure integration of the strategy with EHS research being undertaken nationally and abroad. Ensuring implementation of the strategy and gauging progress in high-priority research also require an assessment of the effectiveness of available mechanisms for interagency collaboration and frequent review of funding needs.

The committee determined that some progress had been made by the NNI in increasing collaborations in EHS research and in tracking how research aligns with its broader goals and strategy. In spite of increased collaboration among federal agencies, the committee did not discern substantial progress toward establishing a mechanism to ensure sufficient management and budgetary authority to develop and implement an EHS research strategy among NNI agencies, and it designated this indicator red. The need for a stronger, convening authority to direct EHS research efforts conducted under the NNI has been similarly raised in several independent reviews of the NNI and its strategy (for example, by the President's Council of Advisors on Science and Technology and the Government Accountability Office).

The committee gave a yellow rating to the extent to which the NNCO is identifying funding needs for collaborative efforts between agencies to accelerate high-priority research progress. To move this indicator toward green will require processes to estimate funding needs periodically and to track and report progress toward meeting the needs.

Providing for Stakeholder Engagement in the Research Strategy

The committee determined that some progress had been made toward actively engaging diverse stakeholders in a continuing manner in all aspects of strategy development, implementation, and revision (indicator yellow). The committee notes recent examples, including the NIOSH-sponsored Safe Nano by Design Conference in Albany, NY, in 2012.

To advance progress in this indicator, the committee considers that additional effort is needed to foster engagement with stakeholders, including supporting the NIOSH forum as an annual event. Similar forums should be created, perhaps around other EHS themes, including consumers, the environment, or the value chain. Such forums could be expanded to standing bodies to ensure continued engagement. In addition, the committee recommends creation of a Stakeholder Advisory Council by NNCO to help to assess the effectiveness of and opportunities for stakeholder engagement.

Conducting and Communicating the Results of Research Funded Through Public–Private Partnerships

Public–private partnerships are needed to expand and enrich EHS research through focused collaborations with stakeholders (for example, ENM manufacturers) and to expand and leverage federal funding. The committee determined that little or no progress had been made in creating well-defined effective partnerships, as measured by execution of partnership agreements, issuance of requests for proposals, and the establishment of a governance structure; it designated this indicator red. NIOSH provides the closest current example: exposure surveys conducted at nanomaterial-manufacturing facilities.

Other examples of public–private partnerships are the European-based Nanotechnology Capacity Building NGOs (NanoCap) that addressed nanotechnology EHS risks and the NNI's signature initiatives[5]. Another blueprint outside the realm of nanotechnology is the Health Effects Institute (HEI); a nonprofit organization chartered to provide science on the health effects of air pollution and funded 50:50 by EPA and the motor-vehicle industry.

Getting to green on the establishment of public–private partnerships may require an approach similar to the model of HEI but with a focus on nanotechnology EHS issues. Critical elements of such a public–private partnership would need to include an independent and accountable governance structure, adequate and shared funding, specific and agreed-on goals, transparent sharing of results and information, and appropriate confidentiality agreements that balance the proprietary needs of industry participants with the public need to share information and make decision-making processes transparent.

Managing Potential Conflicts of Interest

In its first report, the committee noted that the NNI's dual functions—developing and promoting nanotechnology and its applications and mitigating risks arising from such applications—pose tension or even actual conflict between its respective goals. The clearest manifestation of the tension is the disparate allocation of resources between the two functions and the inadequacy of EHS risk research funding. The risks of early-stage technology development are intrinsically riddled with uncertainties; the science needed to provide definitive answers is highly complex and integrative and takes many years to develop. When faced with those nuances, an organization that is evaluated largely according to its success in technology development may not be perceived as able to set EHS research priorities among either resources or study topics effectively.

The committee determined that little progress had been made in establishing a clear separation in management and budgetary authority and accountability between the functions of developing and promoting applications of nanotechnology and understanding and assessing its potential health and environmental implications, and this indicator was designated red. Some progress was made in continued separate tracking and reporting of EHS research activities and funding as evidenced in the research-project funding data in the NNI's EHS research

---

[5]The signature initiatives, although not focused on EHS issues, are collaborations that are intended to spur the advancement of nanotechnology. The NKI is one of the signature initiatives.

strategy and in the NNI's supplement to the president's 2013 budget. This indicator was designated yellow.

The committee maintains that the NNI would benefit from a clearer separation of authority and accountability for its EHS research enterprise in relation to its mandate to promote nanotechnology development and commercialization. But it acknowledges that absent a change in the NNI's statutory mandate, establishment of wholly separate management and budgetary structures and authorities for the dual functions may not be realistic. Nonetheless, other steps could be taken at both the agency level and across the NNI as a whole to address this concern. Agencies should create and adhere to strong scientific-integrity policies governing both intramural and extramural research and should consider creating an ombudsman position to receive, investigate, and resolve complaints or concerns about bias and conflicts of interest related to nanotechnology research. The NNCO should develop and disseminate best practices for identifying, managing, and preventing conflicts of interest and bias in the planning, conduct, and reporting of research.

GOING BEYOND GREEN

Beyond advancing progress on the indicators, the committee projects to a time beyond the domain of its current research recommendations to consider how questions about risk can be best approached in an adaptive and continuing manner so as to update priorities for research and identify concerns.

The committee has repeatedly concluded that more engaged and broadly reaching governance is needed for nanotechnology EHS research. Unlike other "big science" initiatives, such as the Human Genome Project, the applications of nanotechnology permeate every sector of our society and economy; this means that the research spans the missions and jurisdictions of many diverse government agencies and intersects with activities and interests of many stakeholders. Also unlike some initiatives that focus principally or exclusively on technology development and applications, the NNI and its associated agencies are involved in research touching on both applications and implications. Governance processes must actively engage all relevant groups in the process of managing nanotechnology EHS research while addressing perceived or actual conflicts of interest. An integrated and well-coordinated program on both national and global scales would help to ensure that research findings provide the evidence needed to inform EHS decisions so that risks can be effectively managed and, ideally, prevented. Such governance requires empowered leadership: if all agencies are responsible, to some degree, for nanotechnology EHS research, no single agency can be held clearly accountable for its management and progress. The gap in empowered nanotechnology EHS research leadership at the federal level has made coordination and communication challenging and left the enterprise open to perceptions of conflicts between technology development and risk-related research. The committee considers that progress could be accelerated if one of the NNI agencies that has EHS in its mission were designated as the lead agency for directing EHS research throughout the federal government. Alternatively, a new entity could serve that function.

Whatever organization oversees the nanotechnology EHS research strategy, among its most important functions will be to secure and maintain adequate funding for the program, inasmuch as the research strategies outlined by the NNI and the present committee cannot be accomplished without a sustained commitment over at least the next decade. In addition to funding, it is critical that the best researchers nationally and abroad be engaged in this effort and that incentives be established to encourage joint planning and information exchange to address the multidisciplinary research.

An essential element of effective governance and sustenance of the research is a means of ensuring that all stakeholders have access to the growing and evolving body of knowledge—the knowledge commons. Such a resource will provide information relevant to nanotechnology EHS research at multiple levels of detail and thus can improve public understanding, inform policymakers, offer data for future researchers, and shape the focus of future research. For researchers, the knowledge commons will provide access to existing data and will add mechanisms to curate, annotate, and link datasets, so that it will be possible to "bank" the data for consideration by future researchers. The availability of such an inventory would also facilitate oversight of the nanomaterial research program itself and provide greater accountability for research progress. The knowledge commons would provide a context for addressing the recognized need for improved taxonomies of ENM structures, experiments, characteristics, models, effects, and uses. A pragmatic approach would be the development of ontologies that map one set of defined terms onto other commonly used sets to permit data to be fully shared even if researchers adopt different conventions for nomenclature, formatting, and reporting.

CONCLUDING REMARKS

Characterization of the risks posed by ENMs across their life cycles is a scientific challenge that requires integrated, quantitative, and systems-level scientific approaches. It is also an institutional challenge that stretches the conventional roles of agencies and researchers and that looks to how future concerns can be addressed and anticipated. Strong governance is vital if effective, timely, and actionable research is to be ensured. Empowered leadership at the federal level with oversight by a single agency would begin to address many of the organizational barriers. There should be sustained funding for this research and for the infrastructure needed to support data-sharing. The necessary ideal of responsible development of nanotechnology is both daunting and important, but there is no doubt that it is attainable if we plan well for research and for the management of the infrastructure needed to shape and disseminate its findings.

1

Introduction

Despite the increase in funding for research and the rising numbers of peer-reviewed publications over the past decade that address the environmental, health, and safety (EHS) aspects of engineered nanomaterials (ENMs) (NRC 2012; NSET 2012; PCAST 2012), uncertainty about the implications of potential exposures of consumers, workers, and ecosystems to these materials persists. Consumers and workers want to know which of these materials they are exposed to and whether the materials can harm them (see Appendix C). Industry is concerned about being able to predict with sufficient certainty whether products that it makes and markets will pose any EHS issues and what measures should be taken regarding manufacturing practices and worldwide distribution to minimize any potential risk. However, there remains a disconnect between the research that is being carried out and its relevance to and use by decision-makers and regulators to make informed public health and environmental policy and regulatory decisions.

Although those broad topics remain to be better addressed, progress has been made in understanding some aspects of EHS risks posed by ENMs. There is now greater understanding of the dynamic behavior of ENMs; minimum characterization standards, which are still evolving, are now more widely accepted by the field; some reference materials have been distributed and evaluated with models; models for estimating environmental exposures to ENMs have been proposed; and methods for characterizing ENMs in relevant matrices have been developed. However, research on the potential EHS implications of ENMs still lacks context, particularly with regard to future risks, because materials and their uses are changing rapidly. Consequently, the continued focus on available and well-studied materials (such as titanium dioxide) may be misplaced; it is possible that the issues most salient for the future are not being addressed. Some relevant topics have received little attention, such as possible effects of ingested ENMs on human health, measurement of nanoscale characteristics that influence their behavior in situ (for example, the structure of surface coatings), and processes that affect biouptake.

Investments in nanotechnology and the production of ENMs continue to grow; the global market for nanotechnology products is projected to exceed $3 trillion by 2015 (Lux 2008a,b). Industry practices are changing, moving from the use of nanotechnology for enhancement of existing technologies to manufacturing of new products that depend on novel materials and the functionality of nanotechnology (Maynard 2009). Industries are no longer touting nanotechnology initiatives; rather, nanotechnology is becoming embedded in their business practices. However, EHS research efforts are not keeping pace with the evolving applications of nanotechnology, and this issue has motivated development of the research agendas on EHS aspects of ENMs for more than a decade. That context was crucial in the timing of the first report from the present committee, *A Research Strategy for Environmental, Health, and Safety Aspects of Engineered Nanomaterials*, which was released in January 2012, and remains relevant for this second report.

STUDY SCOPE

The US Environmental Protection Agency (EPA) requested that the National Research Council perform an independent study to develop and monitor the implementation of an integrated strategy for research on EHS aspects of ENMs (see Appendix B for complete statement of task). In response to EPA's request, the National Research Council convened the Committee to Develop a Research Strategy for Environmental, Health, and Safety Aspects of Engineered Nanomaterials in 2009. In its first report, as requested, the committee created a conceptual framework for EHS-related research, developed a research plan with short-term and long-term priorities, and estimated resources needed to implement the research plan. For this second report, the committee was tasked with evaluating research progress and updating the research priorities and resource estimates on the basis of results of studies and emerging trends in the nanotechnology industry. Specifically, the committee was asked to address the following:

- What research progress has been made in understanding the environmental, health, and safety aspects of nanotechnology? How does the research progress affect relevance of the initial set of research priorities?
- How have market and regulatory conditions changed and how does this affect the research priorities?
- Are the criteria for evaluating the research progress on the environmental, health, and safety aspects of nanotechnology appropriate?
- Considering the criteria developed, to what extent have short-term and long-term research priorities been initiated and implemented?

Introduction 19

OVERVIEW OF FIRST REPORT

The committee's first report, *A Research Strategy for Environmental, Health, and Safety Aspects of Engineered Nanomaterials* (NRC 2012), presented a strategic approach for developing the science and research infrastructure needed to address uncertainties regarding the potential EHS risks posed by ENMs. The report began by detailing why a research strategy is needed. In describing the rationale for the report, the committee emphasized the complexity of the issues (including the variety of the materials and the applications of materials science), the limitations of the available evidence, and the inadequacy of linkages between current research findings and the evidence needed to prevent and manage potential EHS risks. The committee recognized that there had already been considerable effort in the United States and abroad to identify research needs to support the development and safe use of nanotechnology, especially in the National Nanotechnology Initiative (NNI). Nevertheless, EPA sought to refine existing approaches further.

The first report described a conceptual framework that structured the committee's approach, focusing on emerging ENMs that may pose unanticipated risks and on the influence of properties of ENMs on hazards and exposures (Figure 1-1). The committee then identified critical research gaps that reflected elements of the framework and the tools needed for addressing the gaps. In addition to the conceptual framework and the gaps and tools, the committee identified four broad high-priority research topics that formed the backbone of its proposed research strategy. The committee recognized the evolving nature of ENM research and, in selecting the four broad categories, envisioned a risk-based system that would be informed and shaped by research outcomes and would support approaches to environmental and human-health protection.

The research categories were the following (NRC 2012, pp. 14-15):

- *"Identification, characterization, and quantification of the origins of nanomaterial releases.* Research in this category would develop inventories on ENMs being produced and used, identify and characterize the ENMs being released and the populations and environments being exposed, and assess exposures to measure the quantity and characteristics of materials being released and to model releases throughout their life cycle.
- *"Processes that affect both potential hazards and exposure.* Research topics . . . would include the role of nanoparticle-macromolecular interactions in regulating and modifying nanoparticle behavior on scales ranging from genes to ecosystems; the effects of particle-surface modification on aggregation and nanoparticle bioavailability, reactivity, and toxicity potential; processes that affect nanomaterial transport across biologic or synthetic membranes; and the development of relationships between the structure of nanomaterials and their transport, fate, and effects. As an element of this research category, instrumentation and standard

methods will need to be developed to relate ENM properties to their hazard and exposure potential and to determine the types and extent of ENM transformations in environmental and biologic systems.

- *"Nanomaterial interactions in complex systems ranging from subcellular systems to ecosystems.* . . . Examples of research in this category include efforts to understand the relationships between in vitro and in vivo responses; prediction of system-level effects, such as ecosystem functions (for example, nutrient cycling), in response to ENMs; and assessment of the effects of ENMs on endocrine and developmental systems of organisms.
- *"Adaptive research and knowledge infrastructure for accelerating research progress and providing rapid feedback to advance research.* . . . Activities would include making characterized nanomaterials widely available, refining analytic methods continuously to define the structures of the materials throughout their lifespan, defining methods and protocols to assess effects, and increasing the availability and quality of the data and models. Informatics would be fostered by the joining of existing databases and [the] encouraged and sustained curation and annotation of data."

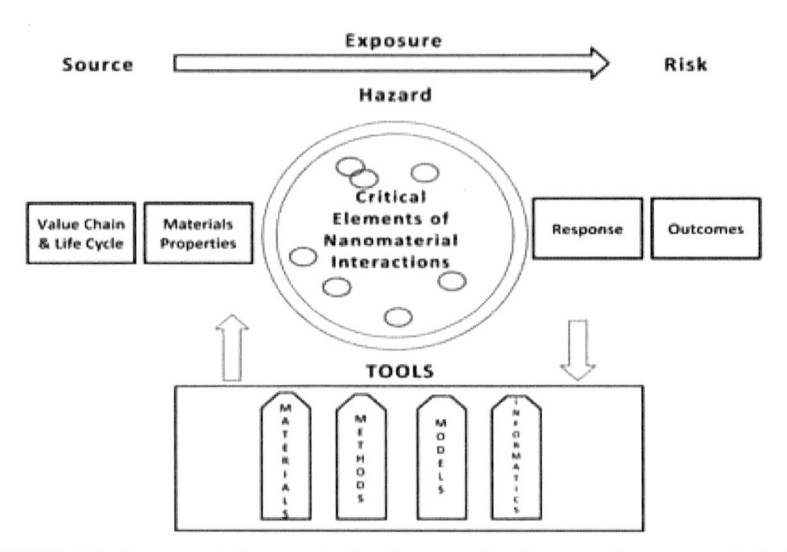

FIGURE 1-1 Conceptual framework for the committee's research strategy depicting "sources of nanomaterials originating throughout the lifecycle and value chain, and therefore the environmental or physiologic context that these materials are embedded in, and the processes that they affect. The circle, identified as 'critical elements of nanomaterial interactions,' represents the physical, chemical, and biologic properties or processes that are considered to be the most critical for assessing exposures and hazards and hence risk" (NRC 2012, p. 55). The lower rectangle "depicts tools needed to support an informative research agenda on critical elements of nanomaterial interactions" (p. 56).

The committee identified financial resources needed to implement research in those categories. In examining resources, it recognized the differential level of research funding for the applications of nanotechnology and the potential implications, but it took a pragmatic approach, recognizing funding constraints, that was centered on current funding levels and informed by expert judgment. The committee recognized a gap between the amount of federal funding and the level of activity required to support the research strategy. It concluded that the core EHS research and development funding[1] by federal agencies should remain constant for at least 5 years because any reduction in funding would be a setback for EHS research. Moreover, additional modest resources from public, private, and international initiatives should be made available for 5 years in five critical categories: informatics ($5 million per year), nanomaterial characterization ($10 million per year), developing benchmark ENMs ($3-5 million per year), characterization of sources ($2 million per year), and development of networks to support collaborative research ($2 million per year). These additional resources would total $22-24 million per year.

The committee discussed the need for mechanisms to ensure implementation of the research strategy and evaluation of research progress. Mechanisms for effective implementation of an EHS research strategy are as essential to the success of the strategy as is the substance of the identified research (NRC 2009). Integration of domestic and foreign participants involved in nanotechnology-related research—including the NNI and federal agencies, the private sector (for example, ENM developers and users), and the broader scientific and stakeholder communities (for example, academic researchers)—was seen as critical for implementation.

Mechanisms identified for implementation included fostering interagency interaction, collaboration, and accountability; developing and implementing mechanisms for stakeholder engagement; advancing integration among sectors and institutions involved in EHS research, such as public–private partnerships; and structural changes that address conflicts of interest.

In considering its task, the committee developed indicators that would serve as criteria for gauging the extent of research and implementation progress in this second report (see Boxes 1-1 and 1-2 for summaries of indicators of research and implementation progress, respectively). Given the short timeframe between the first and second reports, the committee considered that it would be sufficient to anticipate progress in initiating research in each of the four high-priority categories identified and in developing the infrastructure, accountability, and coordination mechanisms needed for implementation of the research strategy. The interval was far too short for substantial new research programs to be in place, let alone for evaluation of research outcomes (NRC 2012).

---

[1]The committee estimated this funding to be about $120 million on the basis of the requested FY 2012 budget. However, the president's 2013 budget revised the 2012 estimate to $102.7 million (NSET 2012).

BOX 1-1 Research-Progress Indicators

Adaptive research and knowledge infrastructure for accelerating research progress and providing rapid feedback to advance the research

- Extent of development of libraries of well-characterized nanomaterials, including those prevalent in commerce and reference and standard materials.
- Development of methods for detecting, characterizing, tracking, and monitoring nanomaterials and their transformations in relevant media.
- Development of methods to quantify effects of nanomaterials in experimental systems.
- Advancement of systems for sharing results of research and fostering development of predictive models for nanomaterial behaviors.
- Extent of joining together of existing databases, including development of common informatics ontologies.

Quantifying and characterizing the origins of nanomaterial releases

Progress indicators will be related to short-term activities:

- Developing inventories of current and near-term production of nanomaterials.
- Developing inventories of intended use of nanomaterials and value-chain transfers.
- Identifying critical release points along the value chain.
- Identifying critical populations or systems exposed.
- Characterizing released materials and associated receptor environments.
- Modeling nanomaterial releases along the value chain.

Processes affecting both exposure and hazard

- Steps taken toward development of a knowledge infrastructure able to describe the diversity and dynamics of nanomaterials and their transformations in relevant biologic and environmental media.
- Progress toward developing instrumentation to measure key nanomaterial properties and changes in them in relevant biologic and environmental media.
- Initiation of interdisciplinary research that can relate native nanomaterial structures to transformations that occur in organisms and as a result of biologic processes.
- Extent of use of experimental research results in initial models for predicting nanomaterial behavior in complex biologic and environmental settings.

Nanomaterial interactions in complex systems ranging from subcellular systems to ecosystems

- Extent of initiation of studies that address heretofore underrepresented fields of research, such as those seeking to relate in vitro to in vivo observations, to predict ecosystem effects, or to examine effects on the endocrine or developmental systems.
- Steps toward development of models for exposure and potential effects along the ecologic food chain.

(Continued)

> **BOX 1-1** Continued
>
> - Extent of refinement of a set of screening tools that reflect important characteristics or toxicity pathways of the complex systems described above.
> - Extent of adaptation of existing system-level tools (such as individual species tests, microcosms, and organ-system models) to support studies of nanomaterials in such systems.
> - Identification of benchmark (positive and negative) and reference materials for use in such studies and measurement tools and methods to estimate exposure and dose in complex systems.[2]
>
> Source: NRC 2012, pp. 181-182.

> **BOX 1-2** Indicators of Progress in Implementation
>
> **Enhancing interagency coordination**
>
> - Progress toward establishing a mechanism to ensure sufficient management and budgetary authority to develop and implement an EHS-research strategy among NNI agencies.
> - Extent to which [the National Nanotechnology Coordination Office] is annually identifying funding needs for interagency collaboration on critical high-priority research.
>
> **Providing for stakeholder engagement in the research strategy**
>
> - Progress toward actively engaging diverse stakeholders in a continuing manner in all aspects of strategy development, implementation, and revision.
>
> **Conducting and communicating the results of research funded through public–private partnerships**
>
> - Progress toward establishment of effective public–private partnerships, as measured by such steps as completion of partnership agreements, issuance of requests for proposal, and establishment of a sound governance structure.
>
> **Managing potential conflicts of interest**
>
> - Progress toward achieving a clear separation in management and budgetary authority and accountability between the functions of developing and promoting applications of nanotechnology and understanding and assessing its potential health and environmental implications.
> - Continued separate tracking and reporting of EHS research activities and funding distinct from those for other, more basic or application-oriented research.
>
> Source: NRC 2012, p. 183.

---

[2]In this report the committee differentiates between benchmark materials and reference materials. Additional details are provided in Chapter 3.

With regard to evaluation of research over the longer term, the committee considered that criteria developed by the National Research Council Committee on Research Priorities for Airborne Particulate Matter[3] (NRC 1998, 1999) should be applied in evaluating research progress periodically. Those criteria are listed below and discussed in more detail in the committee's first report (see NRC 2012, pp. 182-187).

- **Scientific value**: Does the research fill critical knowledge and data gaps?
- **Decision-making value:** Does the research reduce uncertainties and inform decision-making by key stakeholders, for example, decisions about risk assessment and risk management?
- **Feasibility and timing:** Is the research technically and economically feasible, and can it be done in a timeframe responsive to stakeholder and decision-maker needs?
- **Interaction and collaboration:** How well does the research agenda foster the collaboration and interaction needed among scientific disciplines, agencies, academe, and private sector, especially in addressing cross-cutting issues? Are the scientific expertise, capacity, and resources appropriately used to enhance scientific creativity, quality, and productivity?
- **Integration:** How well is the research agenda coordinated and integrated with respect to planning, budgeting, and management, including between government and private organizations?
- **Accessibility:** How well is information about research plans, budgets, progress, and results made accessible to agencies, research organizations, and interested stakeholders?

CONTEXT FOR AND APPROACH TO SECOND REPORT

Several developments during and after completion of the first report influenced the committee's approach to this second report. Notably, the NNI developed and released its own environmental, health, and safety research strategy (NEHI 2011). That strategy builds on previous NNI EHS research-strategy documents (NEHI 2006, 2007, 2008) and helps to develop a framework for coordination among federal agencies and mechanisms to support implementation of the strategy. The committee's original charge to develop and monitor implementation of a research strategy was written in the absence of the 2011 federal EHS research strategy. In addition, there have been other government, academic, industrial, and international efforts, some of which are described in Chapters 2-4 of this report.

---

[3]That committee was asked by Congress to address uncertainties in the scientific evidence related to airborne particulate matter (PM) after the 1997 decision to establish a new National Ambient Air Quality Standard for fine PM.

Introduction 25

Given the short period between the two reports, the committee in this report emphasizes institutional responses to the first report that have implications for conduct of future research. However, considering its charge, the committee assesses the trajectory of progress in the research and implementation indicators identified in the first report while focusing on implementation efforts and tool development necessary to move the research enterprise forward. The committee believes that the indicators remain appropriate for evaluating research and implementation progress.[4] The committee was not able to reevaluate the resource estimates from the first report, as more current funding information was not available.

The committee has developed a graphical construct in Chapter 4 (shown here as Figure 1-2) that complements Figure 1-1 and provides a vision for the EHS nanotechnology research enterprise. Figure 1-2 describes the interrelated and interdependent research activities that are driven by ENM production and highlights the importance of a coordinated research infrastructure.

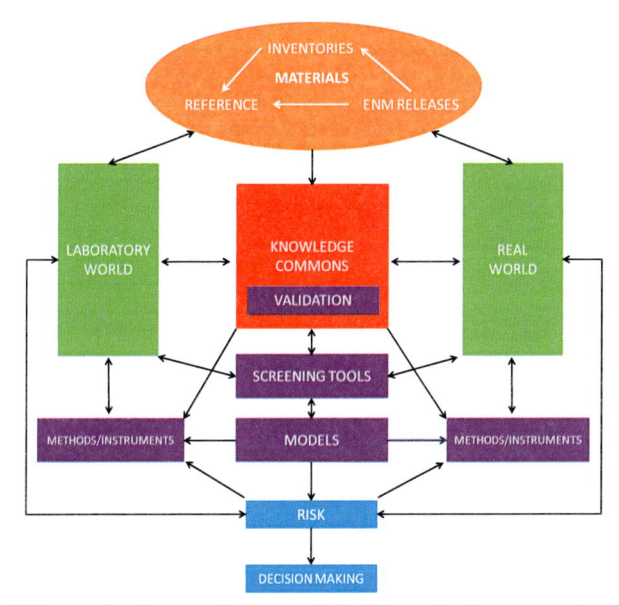

FIGURE 1-2 Nanotechnology environmental, health, and safety research enterprise. The diagram shows the integrated and interdependent research activities that are driven by the production of ENMs. The production of ENMs is captured by the orange oval, labeled "materials", which includes reference materials, ENM releases, and inventories. (An inventory is a quantitative estimate of the location and amounts of nanomaterials produced or current production capacity, including the properties of the nanomaterial.) The knowledge commons (red box) is the locus for collaborative development of methods,

---

[4]In the period between the first and second reports, no substantial changes in market or regulatory conditions that would influence research priorities were noted.

models, and materials, and for archiving and sharing data. The "laboratory world" and "real world" (green boxes) feed into the knowledge commons. The laboratory world comprises process-based and mechanism-based research that is directed at understanding the physical, chemical, and biologic properties or processes that are most critical for assessing exposures and hazards and hence risk (NRC 2012, p. 55). The "real world" includes complex systems research involving observational studies that examine the effects of ENMs on people and ecosystems. The purple boxes capture the range of methods, tools, models, and instruments that support generation of research in the laboratory world, the real world, and the knowledge commons.

As part of its data-gathering efforts, the committee held a workshop on November 7, 2012. The workshop was organized to gain input from federal agencies, researchers, industry, and nongovernment organizations to help in gauging the extent of research progress and understanding efforts that are under way to address scientific uncertainties and research infrastructure needs (see Appendix C for a summary of the workshop). The committee also used its expert judgment based on literature reviews and knowledge of the state of the science to evaluate the extent of research and implementation progress.

Chapter 2 reviews recent reports on EHS aspects of ENMs and the committee's impressions drawn from the workshop. Chapter 3 assesses progress in research and implementation, classifying the research trajectory into three broad categories—substantial progress (green), moderate or mixed progress (yellow), and little progress (red). Chapter 4 analyzes findings from Chapter 3 and suggests pathways for advancing the research enterprise (Figure 1-2). Finally, Chapter 5 considers the overall charge and offers a vision for optimizing the research efforts of the EHS nanotechnology community and provides steps to address the longer-term criteria identified in the committee's first report.

REFERENCES

Lux Research. 2008a. Nanomaterials State of the Market Q3 2008: Stealth Success, Broad Impact. Lux Research, July 1, 2008 [online]. Available: https://portal.luxresearchinc.com/research/document_excerpt/3735 [accessed Mar. 11, 2013].

Lux Research. 2008b. Overhyped Technology Starts to Reach Potential: Nanotech to Impact $3.1 Trillion in Manufactured Goods in 2015. Press release: July 22, 2008 [online]. Available: http://www.nanotechwire.com/news.asp?nid=6340 [accessed Mar. 11, 2013].

Maynard, A.D. 2009. Commentary: Oversight of engineered nanomaterials in the workplace. J. Law Med. Ethics 27(4):651-658.

NEHI (Nanotechnology Environmental Health Implications Working Group). 2006. Environmental, Health, and Safety Research Needs for Engineering Nanoscale Materials. Nanotechnology Environmental Health Implications Working Group, Nanoscale Science, Engineering, and Technology Subcommittee, Committee on Technology, National Science and Technology Council. September 2006 [online]. Available: http://www.nano.gov/NNI_EHS_research_needs.pdf [accessed Mar. 11, 2013].

NEHI (Nanotechnology Environmental Health Implications Working Group). 2007. Prioritization of Environmental, Safety and Health Research Needs for Engineered Nanoscale Materials: An Interim Document for Public Comment. Nanotechnology Environmental Health Implications Working Group, Nanoscale Science, Engineering, and Technology Subcommittee, Committee on Technology, National Science and Technology Council. August 2007 [online]. Available: http://nanotech.law.asu.edu/Documents/2010/08/Prioritization_EHS_Research_Needs_Engineered_Nanoscale_Materials_527_8119.pdf [accessed Mar. 11, 2013].

NEHI (Nanotechnology Environmental Health Implications Working Group). 2008. Strategy for Nanotechnology-Related Environmental, Health, and Safety Research. National Nanotechnology Initiative. Nanotechnology Environmental Health Implications Working Group, Subcommittee on Nanoscale Science, Engineering, and Technology, Committee on Technology, National Science and Technology Council. February 2008 [online]. Available: http://www.nano.gov/NNI_EHS_Research_Strategy.pdf [accessed Mar. 11, 2013].

NEHI (Nanotechnology Environmental Health Implications Working Group). 2011. National Nanotechnology Initiative 2011 Environmental, Health, and Safety Strategy, October 2011. Nanotechnology Environmental Health Implications Working Group, Subcommittee on Nanoscale Science, Engineering, and Technology, Committee on Technology, National Science and Technology Council [online]. Available: http://www.nano.gov/sites/default/files/pub_resource/nni_2011_ehs_research_strategy.pdf [accessed Mar. 11, 2013].

NRC (National Research Council). 1998. Research Priorities for Airborne Particulate Matter. I. Immediate Priorities and Long-Range Research Portfolio. Washington, DC: National Academy Press.

NRC (National Research Council). 1999. Research Priorities for Airborne Particulate Matter. II. Evaluating Research Progress and Updating the Portfolio. Washington, DC: National Academy Press.

NRC (National Research Council). 2009. Review of the Federal Strategy for Nanotechnology-Related Environmental, Health, and Safety Research. Washington, DC: National Academies Press.

NRC (National Research Council). 2012. A Research Strategy for Environmental, Health, and Safety Aspects of Engineered Nanomaterials. Washington, DC: National Academies Press.

NSET (Nanoscale Science, Engineering, and Technology Subcommittee). 2012. The National Nanotechnology Initiative: Research and Development Leading to a Revolution in Technology and Industry: Supplement to the President's FY 2013 Budget. Subcommittee on Nanoscale Science, Engineering, and Technology, National Science and Technology Council. February 2012 [online]. Available: http://www.nano.gov/sites/default/files/pub_resource/nni_2013_budget_supplement.pdf [accessed Mar. 11, 2013].

PCAST (President's Council of Advisors on Science and Technology). 2012. Report to the President and Congress on the Fourth Assessment of the National Nanotechnology Initiative. April 2012 [online]. Available: http://nano.gov/sites/default/files/pub_resource/pcast_2012_nanotechnology_final.pdf [accessed Dec. 5, 2010].

2

Review of Recent Reports and National Research Council Committee Workshop

INTRODUCTION

For its second report, the committee was charged with evaluating research progress since release of its first report and with assessing the extent to which progress has been consistent with its recommendations. Since release of the committee's report in January 2012, a number of national and international efforts have focused on environmental, health, and safety (EHS) aspects of nanotechnology. In the United States, reports have commented on continuing efforts and needs with regard to EHS nanotechnology research, including *The National Nanotechnology Initiative—Supplement to the President's FY 2013 Budget* (NSET 2012) (released in February 2012), *Report to the President and Congress on the Fourth Assessment of the National Nanotechnology Initiative* (PCAST 2012) (released in April 2012), and the Government Accountability Office (GAO) report *Nanotechnology: Improved Performance Information Needed for Environmental, Health, and Safety Research* (released May 2012). In addition, international research efforts directed at EHS aspects of engineered nanomaterials (ENMs) have advanced, particularly in the European Commission (EC) Seventh Framework Program (FP7[1])[2].

In this chapter, the committee reviews findings from key recent reports and assessments and comments on the committee's workshop held in November 2012 (see Appendix C). The chapter is intended to provide insights into the

---

[1] Funding programs created by the European Union to support research. The specific objectives vary depending on the funding period.

[2] The committee recognizes that there are other international research efforts, but this analysis is not intended to be a comprehensive review. Rather it focuses on a few major reports from the US federal government and from the European Union.

broader "systems" of research on EHS aspects of ENMs and to set out a background for Chapters 4 and 5, where the committee offers recommendations for building a more cohesive research enterprise on ENMs and human health and ecosystems. The findings of the recent reports of the US agencies complement the committee's review, and the research efforts in Europe are an important component of the global research enterprise.

THE NATIONAL NANOTECHNOLOGY INITIATIVE SUPPLEMENT TO THE PRESIDENT'S FY 2013 BUDGET

The National Nanotechnology Initiative: Supplement to the President's FY 2013 Budget (NSET 2012) serves as the annual report on the National Nanotechnology Initiative (NNI) and summarizes NNI activities for 2011 and 2012 and plans for 2013. It first examines changes in the balance of investment by program component area (PCA)[3] and then progress toward achieving NNI goals. The focus of this committee is on PCA 7 (EHS) and Goal 4, "Supporting responsible development of nanotechnology". The report details a large number of agency contributions and coordination activities among the federal agencies and international partners that support the EHS research enterprise.[4] A few are highlighted here.

The Consumer Product Safety Commission (CPSC) and the Food and Drug Administration joined the NNI budgeting process in 2011. CPSC has been collaborating with other federal agencies—such as the National Science Foundation and the Environmental Protection Agency (EPA)—to support the development of exposure and risk assessments of nanomaterials and to allow for updates to flag reports of incidents that involve nanotechnology and consumer products (NSET 2012, p. 14). EPA's nanotechnology resources were expected to increase by $1.9 million from 2011 to 2013, with increased efforts focused on nanomaterials that are more environmentally sustainable. EPA proposed to investigate how nanomaterial physicochemical properties influence fate and effects and to couple this research with that on sustainable chemistry and life-cycle assessment. It recently released two requests for applications on sustainable molecular design and synthesis and characterization of chemical life cycle. NIOSH anticipated increasing its investment on three topics in 2013: applying prevention through design principles in its work, developing and sharing containment and control strategies to support responsible development of nanomaterial-based products, and expanding data on worker exposure and health issues in high-volume nanomaterial industries and applications (for example, carbon nanotubes, titanium dioxide, and nanosilver). The National Institute of Standards and

---

[3]Program component area is one of the means by which NNI research and major activities are grouped.

[4]At the time of this writing, the FY 2013 federal budget has not been finalized, and federal agencies are operating under a continuing resolution that will probably affect expected programmatic changes for NNI-funded EHS research.

Technology (NIST) 2013 budget was expected to triple from 2011 levels with increased support for development of measurement methods and standards for detecting and characterizing ENMs and for development of standard reference materials, measurement protocols, and predictive models. NIST released the first reference material for single-walled carbon nanotube soot and plans to release additional nanoscale reference materials (carbon nanotubes, titanium dioxide, silver nanoparticles, and nanoporous glass). The National Institute of Environmental Health Sciences intends to continue investments in its Centers for Nanotechnology Health Implications Research Consortium and is evaluating potential research opportunities in susceptibility factors, including underlying disease, genetic factors, and age.

With regard to EHS research coordination-related activities, CPSC signed an interagency agreement with EPA in 2011 to support research with agencies in the United Kingdom to study potential human exposures to ENMs from consumer products and some environmental sources. In another effort, under the leadership of the International Life Sciences Institute Research Foundation's Nanorelease Project, agencies of the NNI are working with nonprofit groups, industry, and international organizations to develop methods for measuring the release of ENMs from consumer materials (ILSI 2012). EPA researchers and regulators are continuing their collaboration with other federal agencies and nations in the international testing program on nanomaterials under the auspices of the Organisation for Economic Co-operation and Development (OECD) Working Party on Manufactured Nanomaterials. EPA is also partnering with other federal agencies of the NNI in the United States-European Union (EU) collaboration to develop communities of EHS nanotechnology research.

The NNI's progress in responding to recommendations from the President's Council of Advisors on Science and Technology (PCAST 2010) is also detailed, and issues relevant to the work of the present committee are discussed in Chapter 3. With regard to the committee's first report, the Nanoscale Science, Engineering, and Technology (NSET) Subcommittee of the National Science and Technology Council's Committee on Technology (NSET 2012) states that the "NNI agencies are just beginning to assess the first [National Research Council committee] report and consider how its recommendations may be applied to the NNI EHS research program" (p. 61).

THE REPORT TO THE PRESIDENT AND CONGRESS ON THE FOURTH ASSESSMENT OF THE NATIONAL NANOTECHNOLOGY INITIATIVE

The Report to the President and Congress on the Fourth Assessment of the National Nanotechnology Initiative (PCAST 2012) is the fourth review of the NNI by PCAST. Although focused on the whole of the NNI, the report provides some key recommendations regarding EHS research. The report follows up on the recommendations that PCAST made to the NNI in 2010. PCAST acknowledges that the NSET Subcommittee responded to its 2010 recommendations (PCAST 2010) by creating an EHS research strategy and establishing the position of NNI EHS coordinator as a central facilitator among the NNI agencies and international partners. However, it expressed concern regarding the lack of integration between nanotechnology-related EHS research funded through the NNI and information needed by policy-makers to manage potential risks posed by ENMs (PCAST 2012, p. vi). To address that concern, PCAST recommended that "the NSET should establish high-level, cross-agency authoritative and accountable governance of Federal nanotechnology-related EHS research so that the knowledge created as a result of Federal investments can better inform policy makers" (PCAST 2012, p. viii). PCAST also called for an "increase [in] investment in cross-cutting areas of EHS [research] that promote knowledge transfer such as informatics, partnerships, and instrumentation development" (p. viii). The latter recommendation comes from the present committee's 2012 conclusion that an additional $20–25 million was needed for this cross-cutting research that would not undercut other fields of research. PCAST acknowledged the progress made in multistakeholder and interagency collaborations but called for additional coordination particularly in occupational safety and health.

Other subjects that PCAST commented on that are pertinent to EHS include recognition of the "significant hurdles to an optimal structure and management" of the NNI (p. 17). Specifically, the hurdles include "the level of authority that representatives appointed to NSET have within their home agencies to influence the budget allocations needed to meet NNI objectives, the inadequacy of mechanisms to solicit and act upon advice from outside of government, and the level of funding and capacity of the NNCO [National Nanotechnology Coordination Office] leadership to support the agencies in implementing programs that align with the NNI strategic plan" (p. 17). PCAST also commented on the lack of metrics for assessing the effects of federal investment in nanotechnology and stated that "the NNCO should track the development of metrics for quantifying the Federal nanotechnology portfolio and implement them to assess NNI outputs" (p. 21). Many of the PCAST recommendations are consistent with those found in the present committee's first report (NRC 2012).

GOVERNMENT ACCOUNTABILITY OFFICE REPORT, NANOTECHNOLOGY: IMPROVED PERFORMANCE INFORMATION NEEDED FOR ENVIRONMENTAL, HEALTH, AND SAFETY RESEARCH

In May 2012, GAO issued its most recent report to the chairman of the US Senate Committee on Environment and Public Works. The report, *Nanotechnology: Improved Performance Information Needed for Environmental, Health, and Safety Research,* responds to a request to review federal nanotechnology EHS research and examines changes in federal funding for such research, nanomaterials that NNI member agencies focused on in their EHS research in FY

2012, collaboration of NNI member agencies with stakeholders, and the extent to which NNI strategy documents address desirable characteristics of national strategies (GAO 2012, p. 1).

In preparing the report, GAO found substantial increases in funding by NNI agencies for nanotechnology EHS research. In the five fiscal years beginning in 2006, funding for EHS research more than doubled, according to agency reports. Nonetheless, GAO found it difficult to confirm that all the reported projects were focused on EHS research and struggled with the nonuniform reporting approaches used by NNI agencies. Regarding the former issue, GAO reported that "of the 236 projects that the seven agencies reported to us as EHS research for fiscal year 2010, we determined that, for 43 projects (18 percent), it was not clear that the projects met the definition for PCA 7—research primarily directed at the EHS impacts of nanotechnology development and corresponding risk assessment, risk management, and methods for risk mitigation" (p. 18). Those projects accounted for more than $15 million in reported EHS funding or 18% of the total projects. The latter issue identified in the report, nonuniformity of reporting approaches, had been raised by GAO in 2008 and was the subject of one of its recommendations for improvement.[5] In addition, GAO noted that agencies were focusing on limited categories of nanomaterials (primarily carbon nanotubes, nanosilver, and nanoscale titanium dioxide). The report noted that the 2011 NNI EHS research strategy provides an approach to setting priorities among nanomaterials for EHS research, although it commented that it was too early to determine the influence of the approach on the agencies' research.

The 2012 GAO report states that "NNI agencies have collaborated extensively on EHS research and strategies" and have initiated numerous formal collaborative EHS research projects. GAO further reported that "nonfederal stakeholders who responded to GAO's Web-based questionnaire on nanotechnology EHS research" said "that they benefited from collaboration with the NNI member agencies" (GAO 2012, p. 1). Three types of collaborations were identified as the most frequent: "joint data gathering and sharing, joint research solicitations or funding of research consortia, and competitive grants" (p. 34). The questionnaire also identified a "lack of funding and limited awareness" of opportunities for collaboration for some NNI agencies as continuing challenges (p. 1). GAO (2012) comments that despite those challenges, "most respondents rated the 2011 NNI EHS research strategy as somewhat or very effective at addressing nanotechnology EHS research needs" (GAO 2012, p. 1).

Focusing on the 2011 NNI strategic plan (NSET 2011), the 2011 NNI EHS research strategy (NEHI 2011), and the NNI supplement to the president's 2012 budget (NSET 2012), GAO (2012) found that the NNI's EHS program had ad-

---

[5]GAO (2008) recommended "that the Director, OSTP, in consultation with the Director, NNCO, and the Director, OMB [Office of Management and Budget], provide better guidance to agencies regarding how to report [nanotechnology EHS] research" (p. 30). However, GAO (2012) states that "as of February 2012, updated guidance had not been issued" (p. 20).

dressed or partially addressed all six characteristics of what GAO identified as desirable characteristics of a national strategy. The GAO was particularly positive about how the three strategy documents address the first two criteria: purpose, scope, and methodology and problem definition and risk assessment. For desirable characteristic 3 (goals, subordinate objectives, activities, and performance measures), GAO suggests that additional work is needed to articulate priorities, milestones, or outcome-related performance measures that can be used to measure the effectiveness of implementation of an EHS strategy. The 2012 GAO report comments that "independent reviews of the prior NNI strategy documents also noted an absence of performance information" (p. 46). (This finding is also reflected in PCAST 2012 [noted above], regarding the lack of metrics for assessing the effects of federal investments in nanotechnology.) With respect to the fourth and fifth characteristics, GAO's assessment was that the strategy documents had partially addressed resources, investments, and risk management and organizational roles, responsibilities, and coordination (p. 47). However, concerns were raised, because, although "the 2011 NNI EHS research strategy identifies research goals, . . . it is up to the agencies to determine how their funding should be spent" (p. 48). Consequently, there is a perceived lack of oversight of agency roles and little discussion of how agencies will be held accountable for the goals and research needs of the NNI strategy documents. GAO (2012) suggests that "the NNI strategy documents . . . partially address the sixth characteristic describing integration and implementation" (p. 48). This concern arises because the strategy documents do not discuss agency-level EHS research strategies and efforts to map agency strategies to the NNI-level documents are not publically available.

The 2012 GAO report made two recommendations to the director of the Office of Science and Technology Policy (OSTP). It has recommended that "the Director of OSTP coordinate development by the NNI member agencies of performance measures, targets, and time frames for nanotechnology EHS research that align with the research needs of the NNI, consistent with the agencies' respective statutory authorities, and include this information in publicly available reports" (p. 51). In addition, it recommends that "to the extent possible, the Director of OSTP coordinate the development by the NNI member agencies of estimates of the costs and types of resources necessary to meet the EHS research needs" (p. 52).

In summary, as illustrated above with examples from several recent reports, a number of consistent themes have emerged. They include the need for rigor in identifying the most critical questions to be addressed by federal funding through cooperative efforts and with stakeholder engagement. Increased networking among all sectors of the scientific community should be sought. Standards for analysis and reference materials will be critical for this effort; the use of uniform terminology, data descriptions, and approaches to data capture will underpin this broader engagement. Production of not just data but knowledge that can be applied in the construction of decision-support tools and risk assessments will be needed to inform decision-making around EHS issues as we move toward the future. In Chapter 4 of this report, the committee presents a diagram for the EHS nanotechnology research enterprise that builds on those characteristics. It describes the interrelated and interdependent aspects of the enterprise. Although aspirational and relatively simple, it is founded on the key principles for a successful EHS research program that are articulated in the three reports described above and the first report of the present committee.

EUROPEAN UNION EFFORTS

Research on nanotechnology funded through the EC—including EHS research—has been guided since 2004 by a broad strategy. Published in 2004, the *Communication from the Commission: Towards a European Strategy for Nanotechnology* (EC 2004, pp. 21-22) outlined key elements of research investment related to commercial and societal progress. Actions toward identifying and addressing potential human and environmental risks included

- Identifying and addressing safety concerns at the earliest possible stage.
- Reinforcing support for the integration of health, environmental, risk, and other related aspects into research and development (R&D) activities.
- Supporting the generation of toxicology and ecotoxicology data (including dose–response information) and the evaluation of potential human and environmental exposure.
- Adjustment, if necessary, of risk-assessment procedures to account for issues associated with nanotechnology applications.
- Application of risk assessment to consumers, workers, and the environment at all stages of the life cycle of ENMs (including design, R&D, manufacturing, distribution, use, and disposal).

The strategy was influential in guiding ENM safety projects funded under the current and previous research framework programs (FP6 and FP7).

The first implementation report on the strategy, published in 2007 (EC 2007), highlighted a number of steps toward addressing potential risks of nanotechnologies. The steps included expanding the pan-European research program, work by the European Joint Research Center on harmonized methods of characterizing and evaluating the toxicity of ENMs, scientific reviews of research needs and opportunities by the Scientific Committee on Emerging and Newly Identified Risks, and a focus on regulatory review. A number of international collaboration initiatives with the OECD Working Party on Manufactured Nanomaterials, the International Organization for Standardization (ISO), and specific US federal agencies were also highlighted.

The second implementation report on the strategic plan (EC 2009) also emphasizes those themes. Specifically, the EC concluded that from a regulatory perspective there was an urgent need for more action on increasing and consolidating risk-related research funding to keep pace with the development and marketing of new applications; adjusting, validating, and harmonizing available methods for risk assessment for ENMs to ensure the generation of relevant data; improving, developing, and validating methods for characterization, exposure assessment, hazard identification, life-cycle assessment, and simulation, including research on fundamental interactions of ENMs with living organisms; developing suitable reference ENMs for methods development, validation, and quality assurance; developing public databases to serve in the safety assessment of ENMs; and increasing the development of test guidelines and standards within OECD, ISO, and the Comité Européen de Normalisation.

The EC also has published two regulatory reviews on nanosciences and nanotechnologies—the first in 2008 (EC 2008) and the second in 2012 (EC 2012). On the basis of a number of pan-European reviews and analyses of the state of the science and its relevance to regulation, the review concluded that (EC 2012, p. 11)

> In the light of current knowledge and opinions of the EU Scientific and Advisory Committees and independent risk assessors, nanomaterials are similar to normal chemicals/substances in that some may be toxic and some may not. Possible risks are related to specific nanomaterials and specific uses. Therefore, nanomaterials require a risk assessment, which should be performed on a case-by-case basis, using pertinent information. Current risk assessment methods are applicable, even if work on particular aspects of risk assessment is still required.
>
> The definition of nanomaterials will be integrated in EU legislation, where appropriate. The Commission is currently working on detection, measurement and monitoring methods for nanomaterials and their validation to ensure the proper implementation of the definition.
>
> Important challenges relate primarily to establishing validated methods and instrumentation for detection, characterization, and analysis, completing information on hazards of nanomaterials and developing methods to assess exposure to nanomaterials.

In 2004, an EC project was funded to coordinate activities between researchers working on the responsible development of ENMs. NanoImpactNet (NanoImpactNet 2013) ran from 2004 to 2012 and was highly influential in achieving coordination among research groups working on FP6 and FP7 projects across Europe. The key aims of NanoImpactNet were to facilitate collaborations among research projects, communicate results to stakeholders and communicate their needs back to researchers, and help to implement the EC's action plan for nanotechnology. Following in part from NanoImpactNet, all EC research projects addressing the potential risks associated with ENMs are coordinated through the EC NanoSafety Cluster (NanoSafety Cluster 2013), an EC initiative aimed at ensuring strong strategic synergy in the field of EHS nanotechnology research.

The EC NanoSafety Cluster is designed "to maximise the synergies between the existing FP6 and FP7 projects addressing all aspects of nanosafety including toxicology, ecotoxicology, exposure assessment, mechanisms of interaction, risk assessment and standardisation" (NanoSafety Cluster 2013). The objectives "are to facilitate the formation of a consensus on nanotoxicology in Europe; to provide a single voice for discussions with external bodies; to avoid duplicating work and improve efficiency; to improve the coherence of nanotoxicology studies and harmonize methods; to provide a forum for discussion, problem-solving, and planning of R&D activities in Europe; and to provide industrial stakeholders and the general public with appropriate knowledge on the risks to human health and the environment posed by ENMs" (Nanosafety Cluster 2013). Current or completed projects in the cluster represent an R&D investment of about €137 million (about $180 million).

In association with the NanoSafety Cluster, a US–EU discussion on ENM safety research (Finnish Institute of Occupational Health 2012) was formalized in 2011, and there continue to be regular meetings of researchers from both sides of the Atlantic. Through that mechanism, communities of research (CoRs) are being established between the US and the EU. The CoRs are addressing exposure through the life cycle, ecotoxicity testing and predictive models, predictive modeling for human health, databases and ontology, risk assessment, and risk management measures.

In summary, European research on the EHS implications of ENMs has developed into a highly integrated program over the last 8 years. An emphasis on interdisciplinary and interstate collaboration, public–private partnerships, research networks, and integrated programs has contributed to supporting research that is problem-driven and solution-focused. The advantages of that approach are seen in a close integration between research and practice among multiple constituencies. In contrast, the US model of investigator-driven research funded by individual agencies with limited strategic oversight has led to rapid progress in specific fields but less overall coherence than observed in Europe.

Both models have advantages and disadvantages, and there are undoubtedly lessons to be learned on both sides of the Atlantic. As discussed above and as illustrated in Chapter 4, a systematic and networked approach to knowledge creation for improved decision-making would have value around the world. There is considerable opportunity for high-value coordination and integration that can leverage the strengths of both the European and the US efforts to ensure a global strategic research program. This is already beginning to occur through informal and formal collaborations between the US and the EU, but more can be done to ensure efficient and responsive research programs.

NATIONAL RESEARCH COUNCIL COMMITTEE WORKSHOP

On November 7, 2012, the committee held a workshop to obtain input on research progress since release of its first report, *A Research Strategy for Environmental, Health, and Safety Aspects of Engineered Nanomaterials*. An additional focus was on other efforts that were under way to address the scientific uncertainties and research-infrastructure needs for a robust research approach to EHS issues related to ENMs. The information gathered informs the present report. The workshop featured presentations by federal agency and foreign officials, academic researchers, and representatives of nongovernment organizations and industry on the scientific and regulatory framework for EHS research, on recent research progress, and on the applications of the research results to risk management. Panel discussions provided opportunities for expanded dialogue of many of the issues raised during the workshop presentations. A summary of the workshop is provided as Appendix C of this report.

CONCLUSION

Recent reports provide an opportunity to gauge progress on EHS research related to ENMs and on the development of infrastructure for such research. The NNI's supplement to the President's 2013 budget offers an opportunity to review intended enhancements of the NNI program that were developed coincidentally with the publication of the committee's first report. The NNI's supplement to the president's budget does not meet the requirement of completed and published research, but it does provide an opportunity to review the trajectory of NNI work in the context of the progress indicators identified in the committee's first report. Both PCAST (2012) and GAO (2012) provide opportunities to assess the influence of the committee's 2012 report (NRC 2012) on federal oversight groups: PCAST and GAO reinforced many of the committee's recommendations, including the need for clear accountability for NNI spending, particularly on EHS research, for "top-down" strategic direction, and for additional, targeted research funding.

The EC research model aligns more closely with calls for accountability and top-down strategic direction and has been highly successful in stimulating effective research partnerships and integrated approaches to complex challenges. Although there are limitations to that approach, lessons from the EU FP7 program in particular may be usefully applied in the United States. FP7 has been successful in leading to multidisciplinary research programs that are driven by specific safety challenges (for example, the MARINA[6] research program is explicitly focused on developing reference methods that support risk management of engineered nanomaterials), programs that facilitate public–private partner-

---

[6]http://www.marina fp7.eu/.

ships (for example, NANODEVICE[7] brings together researchers and instrument manufacturers to develop new measurement tools), and programs that enable deep cross-disciplinary collaboration and coordination (for example, NanoImpactNet (2013) provides a unique research community–driven forum for information-sharing).

In the committee's November 2012 workshop, it heard from the NNI agencies and the stakeholder communities regarding the progress made in EHS research. The perspective gained there helped the committee in assessing research and implementation progress in Chapter 3 and informed the construction of Figure 4-1. Although the committee recognizes the short timeframe for evaluating research progress, it strongly endorses the concepts of coordinated, transparent efforts and of retrospective impact analysis for assessing progress in advancing knowledge in the EHS nanotechnology research enterprise.

REFERENCES

EC (European Commission). 2004. Communication from the Commission: Towards a European Strategy for Nanotechnology. COM (2004) 338 final. Commission of the European Communities, Brussels. December 5, 2004 [online]. Available: http://ec.europa.eu/nanotechnology/pdf/nano_com_en.pdf [accessed Feb. 27, 2013].

EC (European Commission). 2007. Communication from the Commission to the Council, the European Parliament and the Economic and Social Committee- Nanosciences and Nanotechnologies: An Action Plan for Europe 2005-2009. First Implementation Report 2005-2007. COM(2007) 505 final. Commission of the European Communities, Brussels. September 6, 2007 [online]. Available: http://eur-lex.europa.eu/LexUriServ/LexUriServ.do?uri=COM:2007:0505:FIN:EN:PDF [accessed Feb. 27, 2013].

EC (European Commission). 2008. Communication from the Commission to the European Parliament, the Council and the Economic and Social Committee: Regulatory Aspects of Nanomaterials. COM(2008) 366 final. Commission of the European Communities, Brussels. June 17, 2008 [online]. Available: http://ec.europa.eu/nanotechnology/pdf/comm_2008_0366_en.pdf [accessed Feb. 27, 2013].

EC (European Commission). 2009. Communication from the Commission to the Council, the European Parliament and the Economic and Social Committee- Nanosciences and Nanotechnologies: An Action Plan for Europe 2005-2009. Second Implementation Report 2007-2009. COM(2009)607 final. Commission of the European Communities, Brussels. October 29, 2009 [online]. Available: http://eur-lex.europa.eu/LexUriServ/LexUriServ.do?uri=COM:2009:0607:FIN:EN:PDF [accessed Feb. 27, 2013].

EC (European Commission). 2012. Communication from the Commission to the European Parliament, the Council and the Economic and Social Committee: Second Regulatory Review on Nanomaterials. COM(2012) 572 final. Commission of the European Communities, Brussels. October 3, 2012 [online]. Available: http://eur-lex.europa.eu/LexUriServ/LexUriServ.do?uri=COM:2012:0572:FIN:en:PDF [accessed Feb. 27, 2013].

---

[7]http://www.ttl.fi/partner/nanodevice/Pages/default.aspx.

Finnish Institute of Occupational Health. 2012. EU-U.S. nanoEHS Community of Research (CORs) Flyer [online]. Available: http://www.ttl.fi/en/international/conferences/senn 2012/senn2012_programme/Documents/COR_flyer.pdf [accessed Feb. 1, 2013].

GAO (U.S. Government Accountability Office). 2008. Nanotechnology: Better Guidance is Needed to Ensure Accurate Reporting of the Federal Research Focused on Environmental, Health, and Safety Risks. GAO-08-402. Washington, DC: U.S. Government Accountability Office [online]. Available: http://www.gao.gov/new.items/d08402.pdf [accessed Dec. 5, 2012].

GAO (U.S. Government Accountability Office). 2012. Nanotechnology: Improved Performance Information Needed for Environmental, Health, and Safety Research. GAO-12-427. Washington, DC: U.S. Government Accountability Office [online]. Available: http://www.gao.gov/assets/600/591007.pdf [accessed Dec. 5, 2012].

ILSI (International Life Sciences Institute). 2012. NanoRelease Consumer Products [online]. Available: http://www.ilsi.org/ResearchFoundation/Pages/NanoRelease1.aspx [accessed Jan. 31, 2013].

NanoImpactNet. 2013. European Network on the Health and Environmental Impact of Nanomaterials [online]. Available: http://www.nanoimpactnet.eu/ [accessed Jan. 6, 2013].

NanoSafety Cluster. 2013. Cluster Projects [online]. Available: http://www.nanosafetycluster.eu/ [accessed Jan. 6, 2013].

NEHI (Nanotechnology Environmental Health Implications Working Group). 2011. National Nanotechnology Initiative 2011 Environmental, Health, and Safety Strategy, October 2011. Nanotechnology Environmental Health Implications Working Group, Subcommittee on Nanoscale Science, Engineering, and Technology, Committee on Technology, National Science and Technology Council [online]. Available: http://www.nano.gov/sites/default/files/pub_resource/nni_2011_ehs_research_strategy.pdf [accessed Dec. 27, 2012].

NRC (National Research Council). 2012. A Research Strategy for Environmental, Health, and Safety Aspects of Engineered Nanomaterials. Washington, DC: National Academies Press.

NSET (Nanoscale Science, Engineering, and Technology Subcommittee). 2011. The National Nanotechnology Initiative Strategic Plan. Subcommittee on Nanoscale Science, Engineering, and Technology, Committee on Technology, National Science and Technology Council. February 2011 [online]. Available: http://www.nano.gov/sites/default/files/pub_resource/2011_strategic_plan.pdf [accessed Dec. 20, 2012].

NSET (Nanoscale Science, Engineering, and Technology Subcommittee). 2012. The National Nanotechnology Initiative: Research and Development Leading to a Revolution in Technology and Industry: Supplement to the President's FY 2013 Budget. Subcommittee on Nanoscale Science, Engineering, and Technology, National Science and Technology Council. February 2012 [online]. Available: http://www.nano.gov/sites/default/files/pub_resource/nni_2013_budget_supplement.pdf [accessed Nov. 27, 2012].

PCAST (President's Council of Advisors on Science and Technology). 2010. Report to the President and Congress on the Third Assessment of the National Nanotechnology Initiative. March 2010 [online]. Available: http://www.whitehouse.gov/sites/default/files/microsites/ostp/pcast-nano-report.pdf [accessed Dec. 20, 2012].

PCAST (President's Council of Advisors on Science and Technology). 2012. Report to the President and Congress on the Fourth Assessment of the National Nanotechnology Initiative. April 2012 [online]. Available: http://nano.gov/sites/default/files/pub_resource/pcast_2012_nanotechnology_final.pdf [accessed Dec. 5, 2010].

3

Assessment of Progress

INTRODUCTION

The committee's first report identified indicators of research progress and implementation that could be used as benchmarks for gauging the extent of research and implementation in response to the report. In developing the indicators, the committee acknowledged that given the short timeframe between that report and this second one, there would not be measurable, long-term progress that could be assessed with the indicators. It considered, however, that there would be ample time for initiation of research and for initial development of the infrastructure needed for implementing the research strategy.

In examining the extent of progress that has occurred, the committee is aware that many concomitant environmental, health, and safety (EHS) nanotechnology reviews and planning efforts have occurred within the same period as its own work, including publication of the National Nanotechnology Initiative (NNI) EHS research strategy, other government assessments, international initiatives, and continuing research efforts in general (see Chapter 2). It is neither possible nor useful to try to attribute progress to any particular effort, including this committee's first report. Rather, we examine the trajectories of research and implementation to gauge whether steps have been made toward addressing the indicators identified by the committee and, if not, what efforts are needed to achieve progress.

The committee used a color scheme for categorizing progress: green for substantial progress, yellow for moderate or mixed progress, and red for little progress. It adopted that qualitative approach as suitable for gauging progress given the scope and types of information available. It classified progress on the basis of a consensus of the committee. The assessment considered new activities since preparation of the committee's first report and the trajectory of research progress. Thus, green implies that there are new activities and that sustained progress can be expected, red refers to a situation of limited activity and little expectation of change, and yellow refers to mixed scenarios. The committee recognizes that its assessment is not an exhaustive compilation and evaluation of progress, rather it is intended to provide illustrative examples of progress. Chapter 4, "Getting to Green", describes additional efforts and the pathways that are needed to achieve progress in the research and implementation indicators identified by the committee in the context of the vision for the EHS nanotechnology research enterprise (Figure 1-2).

The discussion below addresses advances made with regard to research and implementation progress indicators identified in the first report. The committee considers that the indicators remain appropriate for evaluating progress. However, in certain cases (as noted), it has clarified the wording or modified the order of the indicators. Boxes 3-1 and 3-2 summarize the indicators, including the committee's assessment of progress—green, yellow, or red. The following text identifies the indicators, discusses progress, and presents the rationale for selection of a particular assessment.

BOX 3-1 Status of Indicators of Research Progress[1]

Adaptive Research and Knowledge for Accelerating Research Progress and Providing Rapid Feedback to Advance the Research

- Extent of development of libraries of well-characterized nanomaterials, including those prevalent in commerce and reference and standard materials
- Development of methods for detecting, characterizing, tracking, and monitoring nanomaterials and their transformations in simple, well-characterized media
- Development of methods to quantify effects of nanomaterials in experimental systems
- Extent of joining of existing databases, including development of common informatics ontologies
- Advancement of systems for sharing the results of research and fostering development of predictive models of nanomaterial behaviors

Quantifying and Characterizing the Origins of Nanomaterial Releases

- Developing inventories of current and near-term production of nanomaterials
- Developing inventories of intended uses of nanomaterials and value-chain transfers
- Identifying critical release points along the value chain
- Identifying critical populations or systems exposed
- Characterizing released materials in complex environments
- Modeling nanomaterial releases along the value chain

(Continued)

---

[1]The wording and ordering of some indicators have been modified from NRC (2012, pp. 181-182). Details of the modifications are noted in the descriptions of the indicators in this chapter.

Assessment of Progress 43

> **BOX 3-1** Continued
>
> **Processes That Affect Both Exposure and Hazard**
>
> - Steps taken toward development of a knowledge infrastructure able to describe the diversity and dynamics of nanomaterials and their transformations in complex biologic and environmental media
> - Progress in developing instrumentation to measure key nanomaterial properties and changes in them in complex biologic and environmental media
> - Initiation of interdisciplinary research that can relate native nanomaterial structures to transformations that occur in organisms and as a result of biologic processes
> - Extent of use of experimental research results in initial models for predicting nanomaterial behavior in complex biologic and environmental settings
>
> **Nanomaterial Interactions in Complex Systems Ranging from Subcellular Systems to Ecosystems**
>
> - Extent of initiation of studies that address the impacts of nanomaterials on a variety of end points in complex systems, such as studies that link in vitro to in vivo observations, that examine effects on important biologic pathways, and that investigate ecosystem effects
> - Extent of adaptation of existing system-level tools (such as individual species tests, microcosms, and organ-system models) to support studies of nanomaterials in such systems
> - Development of a set of screening tools that reflect important characteristics or toxicity pathways of the complex systems described above
> - Steps toward development of models for exposure and potential ecologic effects
> - Identification of benchmark (positive and negative) and reference materials for use in studies and measurement tools and methods to estimate exposure and dose in complex systems

INDICATORS OF RESEARCH PROGRESS

Adaptive Research and Knowledge for Accelerating Research Progress and Providing Rapid Feedback to Advance the Research

In the committee's 2012 report (NRC 2012), the first set of research priorities involved establishing an adaptive infrastructure for research and knowledge generation to accelerate and advance EHS nanotechnology research. The components of this infrastructure include study and reference materials; nanomaterial libraries; instruments and methods for measuring nanomaterials and their transformations; methods or assays to quantify the effects of nanomaterials; databases, ontologies, and tools for sharing research results; and models to uncover relationships among the data. Progress toward those short-term and medium-term research priorities ranged from green for detecting and characterizing engineered nanomaterials (ENMs) in relatively well-characterized media to yellow for development of libraries of well-characterized ENMs, development of methods for quantifying effects of ENMs in experimental systems, and the extent of joining of existing databases, including the elements of an informatics infrastructure. It is expected that the integrated components of the infrastructure will need to be continuously improved to adapt to the growing needs of the research enterprise.

* *Extent of development of libraries of well-characterized nanomaterials, including those prevalent in commerce and reference and standard materials*

BOX 3-2 Status of Indicators of Progress
in Implementation (NRC 2012, p. 183)

Enhancing Interagency Coordination

• Progress toward establishing a mechanism to ensure sufficient management and budgetary authority to develop and implement an EHS research strategy among NNI agencies

• Extent to which the NNCO is annually identifying funding needs for interagency collaboration on critical high-priority research

Providing for Stakeholder Engagement in the Research Strategy

• Progress toward actively engaging diverse stakeholders in a continuing manner in all aspects of strategy development, implementation, and revision

Conducting and Communicating the Results of Research Funded Through Public–Private Partnerships

• Progress toward establishment of effective public-private partnerships, as measured by such steps as completion of partnership agreements, issuance of requests for proposal, and establishment of a sound governance structure

Managing Potential Conflicts of Interest

• Progress toward achieving a clear separation in management and budgetary authority and accountability between the functions of developing and promoting applications of nanotechnology and understanding and assessing its potential health and environmental implications

• Continued separate tracking and reporting of EHS research activities and funding distinct from those for other, more basic or application-oriented research

The committee's first report emphasized that libraries of well-characterized nanomaterials were needed to accelerate EHS nanotechnology research and that the libraries should include nanomaterials that meet the evolving needs of the research community. There has been progress in developing specific nanomaterials that have been appropriately characterized for nanotechnology EHS studies, including gold, silver, and carbon standards developed by the National Institute of Standards and Technology (NIST 2013a), Organisation for Economic Cooperation and Development reference materials characterized by the National Institutes of Health (NIH) Nanotechnology Characterization Laboratory (NCL) for the National Institute of Environmental Health Sciences Nanotechnology Consortium (AZoNano.com 2010), and materials developed in individual research groups and centers. Some of those materials are now available through commercial channels (NanoComposix 2012). However, the composition, structure, properties, impurities, and contaminants of a nanomaterial sample depend on the production, refinement, separation, and purification processes used to make them and can exhibit substantial lot-to-lot variation. In addition, the sample-preparation techniques used for different characterization methods are generally not well documented or reported. For example, the NCL reports (McNeil 2012) that up to 40% of samples submitted to it for characterization were contaminated with endotoxin even though they had been vetted for possible use in therapeutics. It will continue to be difficult to correlate published research results with nanomaterial types unless more detail is provided in publications or documentation of datasets regarding the manufacturing process, lot number, and sample-preparation and characterization methods used.

For the last few years, it has been recognized that nanomaterials for EHS research need to be well characterized in the media in which they are used (Richman and Hutchison 2009; von der Kammer et al. 2012; Pettit and Lead 2013). Although there has been progress in that respect (for example, use of the same well-characterized materials in various studies to allow comparison of results), there still are no recommended standard materials for characterization. Nanomaterials produced for fundamental or applied research are rarely characterized adequately for EHS research. Therefore, new nanomaterials that are produced and developed for applied research typically cannot be used more broadly for EHS research, because of the different types of characterization needed, which depend on the intended uses.

With respect to developing materials libraries to support nanotechnology EHS research, the committee concludes that much work is needed. There has been an emphasis on nanomaterials that have been documented to be most prevalent in commerce—including nanosilver, carbon nanotubes (CNTs), and zinc oxide (ZnO) (OECD 2008; PEN 2013)—although a recent survey of the patent literature suggests that there is probably a more diverse set of materials that are being and will be incorporated into products (Leitch et al. 2012). To accelerate research, a larger set of nanomaterials is needed to identify the structural features responsible for potential biologic and environmental effects. Specifically, ENMs should be selected to address hypotheses regarding the influences of individual structural parameters (for example, surface coating, surface functionality, ion release rates from core material, core sizes, and material purity). Thus far, there has been little progress in producing structurally analogous sets (or libraries) of well-characterized nanomaterials (Harper et al. 2011). As a result, it is not possible to conduct systematic studies of families of structurally related nanomaterials to determine how structure influences effects. Not surprisingly, the structural diversity of the materials that have been produced does not yet support the needed breadth of nanotechnology EHS studies.

Thus, although there has been some progress in producing and characterizing new nanomaterials to support EHS research, there are large gaps, and progress toward this goal is categorized as yellow.

Development of methods for detecting, characterizing, tracking, and monitoring nanomaterials and their transformations in simple, well-characterized media

In its first report, the committee gave high priority to research that promotes development of critical supporting tools, including methods of characterizing how the properties of ENMs affect their interactions with humans and the environment (NRC 2012). Those capabilities need to be developed in the short term and ramped up to become sustainable in the longer term. In simple and relatively well-characterized media (such as deionized water and physiologic buffer with known composition), substantial progress has been made in developing analytic tools and methods for detecting and characterizing nanomaterials. (Detection and characterization of ENMs in more complex environmental media are discussed later in this chapter.) Several agencies—including NIST, the US Army Corps of Engineers Engineer Research and Development Center, and the NCL—have active research programs in place that are aimed at developing and validating the tools (NSET 2012a). Some components of activities in two research centers funded by the Environmental Protection Agency (EPA) and the National Science Foundation (NSF) are aimed at developing and validating ENM detection and characterization methods; in most cases, these are applications of, or adaptations of, existing tools, including x-ray spectroscopy (Ma et al. 2012; Lawrence et al. 2012), spectrometry (Mitrano et al. 2012), and optical methods (Fatisson et al. 2012). Some new methods are being developed to measure important ENM properties, such as surface hydrophobicity of nanoparticles (Xiao and Wiesner 2012) and chirality of single-walled CNTs (Khan et al. 2013). In addition, the nanotechnology EHS research community now recognizes the dynamic nature of nanomaterials and the need to characterize nanomaterial transformations and the transformed materials (Levard et al. 2012; Liu et al. 2012; Lowry et al. 2012a; Nowack et al. 2012).

The committee classifies this indicator as green because of the number of programs initiated or under way in various agencies and the progress evident in the peer-reviewed literature (as described above). However, characterization efforts are generally (not exclusively) limited to studies in well-controlled model media, and more work is needed to extend understanding to more complex systems (discussed later in this chapter). Some ENM properties are still difficult to measure, such as the properties of adsorbed macromolecules and the structure of the outer surface layers of nanomaterials. Techniques for routine monitoring of nanomaterials in environmental media (for example, wastewater treatment-plant effluent) are not available (as discussed later). Finally, although there are many data on ENM characteristics and likely transformations, cross-validation and synthesis of the data to provide *knowledge* about ENM properties and the environmental properties that lead to the transformations have not occurred.

- *Development of methods to quantify effects of nanomaterials in experimental systems*

The committee's first report identified the need for standardized methods for assessing environmental effects of nanomaterials in the environment and the need for markers for assessing toxicity. It also identified a lack of information on effects, especially ecosystem effects, of longer-term nanomaterial exposures of organisms and human populations. Studies have been published on the potential effects of acute nanomaterial exposures of various organisms in aquatic and terrestrial environments. However, it is difficult to integrate the data to develop the information needed to predict the effects of ENMs, because of the lack of standardized assays, the variety of ENMs, the variety of organisms and experimental conditions used, and the fact that many studies have examined primarily acute mortality outcomes. More toxicity information on a greater variety of nanomaterials is needed so that different ENM properties and different end points can be examined. Standardization of assays and development of reference materials for positive and negative controls are also needed to ensure that the data gathered for toxicity assays are comparable and useful.

The EPA, the Food and Drug Administration (FDA), and the National Institute for Occupational Safety and Health (NIOSH) have not identified assays targeted at specific outcomes to assess nanotoxicity. There is a need to standardize toxicity assays, both in vitro and in vivo, to reduce variability within and between laboratories and to improve consistency of results among different laboratories. For example, a round-robin in vitro study involving 10 laboratories in the United States and Europe to characterize nanoparticles before toxicity testing revealed that although there was improved reproducibility between laboratories because of adherence to strict protocols for shipping, measurement, and reporting, measurements of polydisperse suspensions of nanoparticle aggregates or agglomerates were not reproducible (Roebben et al. 2011). The use of ultrasonication increased variability among polydisperse suspensions. With respect to quantifying effects of nanomaterials in vivo, a 2013 round-robin study (Bonner et al. 2013) by four laboratories in the United States investigating pulmonary responses in mice and rats to three forms of nano-titanium dioxide (nano-TiO$_2$) and three forms of multiwalled CNTs (MWCNTs) showed some interlaboratory variability of the inflammatory response to TiO$_2$, but the relative potency of the MWCNTs was similar among all laboratories. Although some agencies, such as NIST, are evaluating different protocols (NIST 2013b), the need for standard operating procedures has not been fully met. Establishing such procedures for all phases of ENM preparation and toxicity testing is required to increase consistency of results among laboratories.

Several studies have identified acute ecotoxic effects of ENM exposures and issues associated with traditional nanotoxicity assays (see Klaine et al. 2008 and above references for review). However, there is little information on effects on ecologically relevant species or on ecosystem-level effects of the chronic low-dose exposures to ENMs that are expected in the environment (Bernhardt et al. 2010; Gottschalk and Nowack 2011). Investigations of perturbations in whole-organism systems are also lacking. Efforts have concentrated on oxidative stress, which may be a fleeting reaction of an organism to ENM exposures and may not be the sole mechanism of effects. The committee's 2012 report called for targeted assays for assessing nanotoxicity. Efforts to assess toxicity by using high-throughput assays at the EPA–NSF funded centers (Lin et al. 2013; Nel et al. 2013) may provide some standard acute-toxicity information on selected nanomaterials. The relevance of those assays to more realistic chronic low-dose exposures and population-level effects has not been established. The committee specifically suggested development of a standard battery of assays and novel assays that may be required to describe the various effects of many types of nanomaterials, including ones that have new biologic activities. Standardized assays for ecosystem effects of even standard chemicals are lacking. The EPA–NSF funded centers may be an indication of support for those types of assays, but this is the only direct support identified for this topic.

The committee considered that there was some research progress in this category, but the progress was marked yellow because of the lack of identification of a set of methods to determine effects. More information on the variety of potential mechanisms and research that elucidates these mechanisms will move this indicator toward green.

Extent of joining of existing databases, including development of common informatics ontologies

Some progress has been made toward the development of informatics ontologies and sharing of databases. For example, the Big Data Initiative was announced in March 2012 "to greatly improve the tools and techniques needed to access, organize, and glean discoveries from huge volumes of digital data" with support from NSF, NIH, the Department of Energy (DOE), the Department of Defense (DOD), the Defense Advanced Research Projects Agency, and the US Geological Survey (OSTP 2012). The new program defines *data* as including data, publications, samples, physical collections, software, and models (NSF

2010). The same comprehensive definition underpins the new NSF Nanotechnology Signature Initiative for a Nanotechnology Knowledge Infrastructure (NKI) with participation by the Consumer Product Safety Commission (CPSC), DOD, DOE, EPA, FDA, the National Aeronautics and Space Administration, NIH, NIOSH, NIST, NSF, and the Occupational Safety and Health Administration (OSHA). In addition, the NKI will support the new Materials Genome Initiative (MGI) (NSET 2012b) so that informatics approaches, data curation workflows, protocols, and standards developed through MGI activities may initially be explored for nanoscale activities by the NKI effort.

Coordination of activities in the United States and the EU has been established through the Communities of Research (CoRs) by the National Nanotechnology Coordination Office (NNCO) and the EU. The CoRs include "predictive modeling for human health, ecotoxicity testing and predictive models, exposure through the life cycle, databases and ontology, risk assessment, and risk management and control" (Finnish Institute of Occupational Health 2012). The ontology CoR is responsible for coordinating informatics needs for all the CoRs, and its databases provide a mechanism for developing prototype systems and applications to support information-sharing, annotation, validation, and curation for experimental, computational, and theoretical efforts in nanotechnology. The EU–US CoRs represent an important opportunity for international collaboration to develop an infrastructure that can serve both communities.

Although those new programs are promising, progress in developing elements of an informatics infrastructure has been less encouraging. The foregoing examples show the need for libraries of nanomaterials; for improved reporting on nanomaterial production processes and sample-preparation techniques; for new methods for characterizing, tracking, and monitoring nanomaterials and their transformations; for methods for quantifying the effects of nanomaterials; and for systems for sharing research results and the development of predictive models for nanomaterial behaviors. Core systems, services, and applications are not yet available or have been insufficiently adopted, and this gap impedes research and the translation of research findings into products. For example, a harmonized nomenclature system that facilitates and informs nanomaterial classification and development does not exist; data and metadata standards are not established; reproducibility of methods (ruggedness testing) has not been established; and the sensitivity data are not shared and therefore cannot be used to improve the reproducibility of methods or to inform error propagation in risk analyses. The same general limitations are present for model development: furnishing accurate nanomaterial and nanoproduct structural models on the appropriate scales; developing and validating the models and their sensitivity to input parameters, computer programs, the choice of run-time parameters, computer architectures, and compilers at the relevant dimensions and time scales; and accessing and validating models for the physical, chemical, and biologic systems of interest, also at the appropriate dimensions and time scales. In that regard, NanoHUB constitutes a substantial and important start, providing a stable code for different users and assuming the burden of hosting the code; providing computers, storage, and user services; archiving and sharing data, metadata, and information about results; and comparison with related model results.

Finally, there is an overarching need for informatics to augment collaboration and accelerate research and translation by facilitating access to data. Examples of the need for informatics include the accelerated adoption of models through NanoHUB and the increased amount of interlaboratory testing of methods by various organizations (NIEHS 2012; ILSI 2013a). There are abundant examples of data that are not available through the publication process and that in many cases are not accessible on any database—such as sensitivity data on methods and validation data on models—but there are several areas of particular interest and activity. For example, high-throughput methods are increasingly used in nanotechnology-EHS research, and applications from EPA–NSF funded centers (Thomas et al. 2011; Mandrell et al. 2012) promise to generate large, correlated datasets obtained with standardized screening methods. ISA-TAB-Nano[2], a new standard for data exchange, is emerging; its harmonized data formats incorporate high-throughput screening assays and methods for nanomaterial characterization. Metadata capture will be possible through the NanoParticle Ontology (NPO) that builds on NIH's Enterprise Vocabulary System. However, most important are the increasing informatics efforts (mentioned above) that promise new support and substantially increased collaboration—the NKI, collaboration with the MGI, and the other NNI signature initiatives, particularly the EU-US CoRs. Those developments collectively signal heightened interest in increasing data quality throughout nanotechnology and nanoscience and heightened activity in establishing a coherent infrastructure for increased collaborative research among all the disciplines.

Additional data inputs are possible if databases are compiled from other studies. One potential mechanism, as mentioned in the committee's first report, is NSF's requirement that all grant proposals include a two-page plan for how data will be managed and shared publicly. However, modifications of that requirement through creation of a data commons could allow the collection of all nanotoxicity data from NSF-funded studies rather than siloed storage and retrieval sites established by each researcher.

On the basis of the still unmet need for more data-integration mechanisms, the committee has characterized this indicator as yellow.

Advancement of systems for sharing the results of research and fostering development of predictive models of nanomaterial behaviors

---

[2]This format is an extension of the Investigation-Study-Assay (ISA) Tabular formats used for genomics and high-throughput screening (for example, MAGE-TAB) and adds a material file to permit transmission, linkage, and provenance of data on the nanomaterial samples being studied. This publication represents an initial step to providing one aspect of the needed infrastructure for sharing research data, and it is not yet clear how it will be received by the research community.

In its first report, the committee identified the need to develop predictive models for ENM behaviors and risk. However, the development of models cannot occur in isolation from data generation. Coordination is needed in the short term to ensure that experimental, modeling, and informatics efforts contribute to a coordinated, functional infrastructure. There is a need to collect, store, archive, and share data related to assessing the potential effects of ENMs (as described in the previous section) so that these data can be used to develop predictive models of ENM behavior. The goals of advancing systems for sharing and developing models of behavior are intimately related in that the models and data structures are both influenced by the specific questions related to exposure to ENMs and the resulting effects that need to be addressed. Therefore, the needs for models and infrastructure to support the models are assessed together.

There has been some progress in development of models to predict nanomaterial exposures and toxicity (Gottschalk et al. 2011; Nel et al. 2013). Several government agencies have instituted specific programs to develop and test different models to assess ENM behavior (for example, fate in the environment, releases from consumer products, plant uptake, and occupational exposure), including EPA, NIST, FDA, DOD, the US Department of Agriculture, and NIOSH (NSET 2012a). Efforts are also in place to develop computational models for toxicity (for example, EPA's ToxCast program). Finally, there has been progress towards the development of empirical predictive models as opposed to fully mechanistic models for behavior (Hou et al. 2013; Westerhoff and Nowack 2013). These models rely on empirical correlations (for example, partition coefficients) rather than complete mechanisms. The models can be developed in less time than fully mechanistic models, and can predict approximate behaviors (for example, in a wastewater treatment plant) and may be used to support regulatory decisions.

The committee classifies progress in this category as yellow because, despite the development and use of the models in the nanotechnology-EHS community, there is not yet a central repository for sharing the models (although NanoHub may be appropriate), and many needed models have not yet been developed, such as models to predict the structure of ENM surfaces in various environments. Most important, there is a paucity of data for calibrating and validating models that have been developed; for example, there are very few data on ENM concentrations and speciation in environmental and biologic media that can be used to calibrate fate and transport or biodistribution models. The absence of metadata and validation data for most models hampers their broad acceptance and use because they are not deemed reliable and accurate.

Some progress is being made in the collection, storage, and archiving of ENM physical and chemical properties. For example, the Nanomaterials Registry (NR) has been developed by the Research Triangle Institute with funding from NIH (Nanomaterialregistry 2013). The NR will provide a curated repository of ENM information (for example, ENM properties) from a wide array of studies that used the materials. The repository would allow researchers to compare model results for behaviors and effects of ENMs by using data on the nanomaterials stored in the NR. Incorporation of information on biologic and environmental interactions in the NR is also being considered. Other databases are being created (for example, the Nano-Bio Interactions Knowledgebase) with similar aims: to capture and store information about nanomaterial properties and behaviors that allow development of structure–activity relationships and other scientific synthesis using large datasets. Finally, the new standard data format, ISA-TAB-Nano, for sharing results obtained with analytic methods for characterization of nanomaterial properties and effects has recently been published (Thomas et al. 2013).

The committee classifies progress in this category as yellow because despite initial efforts and models developed, the models and data are not yet widely available and there is no agreement about the appropriate architecture for the databases, no agreement about ontology (although it is being developed through the NPO), and little discussion of interoperability and sharing among databases. Furthermore, the datasets are sparse, there is not a consistent level of variation in the collected data to allow rigorous scientific synthesis, and the breadth of data and metadata needed to make the datasets useful has not been determined or verified with a realistic "test bed" scenario.

Quantifying and Characterizing the Origins of Nanomaterial Releases

The quantities and characteristics of ENMs produced and the products that they enable influence human and ecosystem exposures. Even a thorough understanding of ENM transport, transformation, and effects is not sufficient to describe the effects of ENMs on human health and ecosystems if little is known about how the materials are produced and emitted and the forms in which they are introduced into the environment. Therefore, inventories[3] are needed that describe what ENMs are being produced, how they are being used, and what their forms are along the value chain. However, the creation of inventories of nanomaterials is based on the notion that there is agreement as to what constitutes a nanomaterial. The committee returns to the issue of defining ENMs in Chapter 5.

Progress in this research priority ranged from yellow to red; no priorities were classified as green. Yellow was the designation given for the extent of progress in developing inventories of ENMs, in identifying critical release points

---

[3]An inventory is a quantitative estimate of the location and amounts of nanomaterials produced or current production capacity, including properties of the nanomaterials produced. Information on the nature of the systems into which nanomaterials might be released during their production and the procedures for manufacturing the ENMs are important for assessing the possible transformations that nanomaterials might undergo and the lifecycle impacts associated with energy and material use and waste generated. A broader definition also includes an enumeration of the amounts and uses of nanomaterials downstream in the value chain (that is, the types of products using nanomaterials, the fraction of ENMs by weight in the products, and the quantities of these products).

Assessment of Progress 53

along the value chain, in identifying critical populations, and in characterizing released materials in complex environments. Because those priorities serve as a prerequisite to model development, the ability to model releases along the value chain was denoted as red.

- *Developing inventories of current and near-term production of nanomaterials*

The committee identified efforts in academic and government laboratories to quantify and characterize the origins of nanomaterial releases and private-sector efforts focused on market reports. Production quantities, estimates of trends in production quantities, and the associated descriptions of what is being produced are components of what is referred to as inventories of nanomaterial production. The examples cited are not meant to be exhaustive but rather to provide evidence that progress is being made. Work on estimating near-term inventories of nanomaterial production of many of the more commonly cited nanomaterials (TiO2, CNTs, fullerenes, nanosilver, and nano-ZnO) at the base of the value chain has already been published by EPA–NSF funded researchers (Robichaud et al. 2009; Hendren et al. 2011). Some of the materials were described by Michael Holman, of Lux Research, in the committee workshop (see Appendix C) as being the most likely to dominate in commercial products in the foreseeable future. Whether that is the case and whether more advanced (for example, hybrid[4]) nanomaterials will grow in importance remain unclear inasmuch as estimates of nanomaterial production are subject to constant change and the uncertainties around production quantities are large. Such inventories are generally snapshots of nanomaterial production at a given time. The number of such inventories is quite small, but a related consideration is the lack of a systematic process that includes mechanisms and incentives for collecting such information; information-management plans for storage, dissemination, and interpretation of the data; and appropriate regulatory infrastructure. Progress in characterizing production amounts of nanomaterials is therefore likely to remain incomplete for some time and has been given an indicator status of yellow.

- *Developing inventories of intended uses of nanomaterials and value-chain transfers*

Research in NIST and EPA–NSF funded centers is quantifying releases of nanomaterials from composite matrices, a likely disposition of many nanomaterials. Those centers are characterizing the release of CNTs, nanoclays, and nanosilver from porous foams and solid polymers through simulated abrasion and in various biologic fluids (Wohlleben et al. 2011; Liu et al. 2012; Nguyen et al. 2012).

---

[4] A hybrid nanomaterial is one that results from combining different nanomaterials to form a new material that has characteristics different from those of the original materials.

Such nano-composite materials impart antimicrobial, strength, or flame-retardant properties to fabrics, foams, and plastics that may be used in consumer products.

Analysis of value-chain transfers of nanomaterials that enter commerce from primary production to integration into a multitude of consumer products is also being conducted in an EPA–NSF funded center and in an NSF-funded center. Such analyses remain inadequate, perhaps because few nanomaterials are widely used in commerce. Given the mixed picture of progress, the committee designated this item as yellow.

- *Identifying critical release points along the value chain*

As discussed in the first report, "each nanomaterial or product containing nanomaterials along the steps of the value chain has an associated life cycle of production, distribution, use, and end-of-life releases that may affect human health and the environment" (p. 56). There has been progress in developing inventories of a small number of key nanomaterials and in mapping key elements of the value associated with a subset of these materials, but actual modeling of releases of nanomaterials to the environment along the value chains does not appear to have been initiated to any important degree. Limited by progress in the prerequisite steps of compiling information on inventories in the value chains highlighted above, identification of likely release points that may result in direct exposure of humans in the workplace or during transportation, use and end-of-use of nanomaterial-containing products, and the associated points of release to ecosystems has not been quantitatively modeled.

Since the preparation of the committee's first report, additional commitments by federal agencies and their collaborators have been identified. Many of those efforts are summarized in the NNI budget supplement for 2013 (NSET 2012a). In 2013, NIST expanded its nanotechnology EHS program to focus on the safe manufacture, use, and disposal of ENM-containing products. Those activities include development of measurement methods and standards to detect ENMs in nanomaterial-enabled products and to assess their releases. NIST has indicated that this work will focus on the ENMs of greatest regulatory interest according to production volume (NSET 2012a, p. 17). Candidates have been reported to include silver TiO_2, cerium oxide, CNTs, and clay-based composites. Release to all environmental media is of interest, but the focus appears to be on airborne releases, with NIST and CPSC implementing multiyear interagency agreements to cooperate in these efforts. EPA also has indicated an expansion of efforts to characterize properties of ENMs in products that affect their release, fate, and transport in the environment. EPA appears to be focusing its efforts on carbon-based, metal-based, and metal oxide–based products. This focus is likely to improve our understanding of the potential for release of ENMs from products throughout the value chain. In support of those efforts, the EPA–NSF funded centers are focused on increased understanding of human exposures to ENMs, including those released from products in commerce. CPSC staff are reportedly also supporting such efforts in the centers. NIOSH and EPA are conducting testing to evaluate release of nanosilver from uses of nanomaterial-containing consumer products. Like NIST, CPSC, and EPA, NIOSH continues its focus on airborne releases of nanomaterials from products. An increasing number of studies are measuring releases of ENMs at manufacturing sites (Tsai et al. 2008, 2009, 2012; Methner et al. 2010; Kuhlbusch et al. 2011); however, there is a lack of data on consumer exposure along the value chain. Chen et al. (2010) simulated human exposure to a TiO_2-containing aerosol in a spray that can be used as a cleaning agent. Federal agencies—including NIST, CPSC, EPA, NIOSH, and OSHA—are collaborating with nonprofit, industry, and international groups under the auspices of the International Life Sciences Institute (ILSI) Research Foundation's Nanorelease Project (ILSI 2013a). In 2013, work on refinement of testing methods is expected to lead to a round-robin approach to testing products for release of ENMs.

Although efforts to address release of ENMs from products are under way, additional efforts will be needed. In particular, the focus on large-production-volume ENMs may limit our ability to assess emerging materials before they enter the marketplace in consumer products. In addition, the focus on aerosol releases provides an incomplete perspective on all pathways of release to the environment. Expansion of these efforts will be critical for the assessment of potential EHS risks posed by ENMs throughout the value chain of nanomaterial-enabled products. Because a more comprehensive and comparative view of where nanomaterials may be released along the value chain is needed to identify where to mitigate risks, the indicator is yellow.

Identifying critical populations or systems exposed

In its first report, the committee noted the importance of characterizing not only the quantity and nature of ENMs to which humans and ecosystems are exposed but possible changes in exposed populations and systems that occur during ENM releases throughout the life cycle and value chain. Understanding the complexity of ecosystems (that is, the interaction of the abiotic and biotic and the variety of environments and organisms) and of human populations (including such factors as age, socioeconomic status, health status, behavior and activities, and exposure pathways) requires an integrative research structure involving collaboration among disciplines and among stakeholders. As a high-priority short-term research goal, the committee has suggested identifying exposed human populations and the magnitude of exposure in different ecosystems after determination of critical release points along the ENM value chain. There has been some research activity but little progress in identifying critical human populations exposed to ENMs. NIOSH is developing public–private partnerships with companies manufacturing ENMs and has conducted exposure assessments at their manufacturing sites (for example, producers of titanium dioxide nanoparticles, CNTs, and carbon nanofibers) (NIOSH 2012a). That activity is a useful start in characterizing released ENMs in workplace environments. However, considerable work is needed to measure exposures throughout the ENM life cycle and value chain. For example, the influence of accumulation along the food chain on exposure and exposure to different types of CNTs during production, distribution, use, and disposal need to be evaluated (Helland et al. 2007).

Some consumer products may be of greater concern than others (for example, cosmetics applied as sprays), given the form of the ENMs within products. Initial efforts by ILSI (2013b) and the EU (Kuhlbusch et al. 2011) are leading to strategies to assess potential ENM exposures from consumer products. Exposures from discarded products after disposal or end-of-life use (for example, from landfills) need to be measured.

With respect to ecosystems, some individual research efforts to examine exposures to ENMs are supported by federal funding. Examples include examination of titanium dioxide in wastewater outputs (Westerhoff et al. 2011), CNTs in aquatic systems (von der Kammer et al. 2012), and movement of ENMs through groundwater (Phenrat et al. 2010; Kim et al. 2012), and research into distribution of ENMs into model ecosystems (Lowry et al. 2012b; Schierz et al. 2012). EPA has also funded several projects to examine movement of ENMs in systems and to develop technologies for detecting nanomaterials (EPA 2012). However, for the majority of ENMs, important questions remain: What is their exposure potential in different environments, such as soil, water (aquifers), the food chain, and wastewater? How do alterations in the chemistry of ENMs influence the potential for ecosystem exposure?

Given the challenge of effectively measuring ENM exposures along the value chain and some, but limited progress in identifying both human populations and ecosystems exposed, the committee has labeled this indicator yellow.

Characterizing released materials in complex environments[5]

Characterization of materials that are released into the environment remains a challenge because released materials are present at low concentrations, are often transformed during release, and must be analyzed within structurally and compositionally heterogeneous matrices (von der Kammer et al. 2012). For example, a nanoparticle released into a waterway may undergo a wide array of transformations that would render it difficult to detect and characterize:

- The nanoparticle becomes highly diluted, and this makes detection and characterization difficult even if it is not transformed.
- The nanoparticle surface coating or core may be fully or partially degraded, and this can result in a complex mixture of *unknown chemicals* that are more difficult to detect and characterize. In addition, it may not be possible to

---

[5]This indicator originally was phrased as "Characterizing released materials and associated receptor environments" (NRC 2012, p. 181).

relate whatever is detected to the primary nanoparticles released and to distinguish between degradation products and naturally occurring nanoscale species.
- The nanoparticle surface may be coated rapidly by natural organic matter or proteins, and this can complicate detection and isolation and make it difficult to characterize the surface chemistry.

Releases have been tracked by monitoring the elemental compositions of macroscopic products or the bulk environments into which nanomaterials are released. Such techniques as inductively coupled plasma mass spectroscopy (ICP-MS) are now widely used to gain information about elemental composition of ENMs in aqueous samples (for example, surface waters) (Heithmar 2011; Mitrano et al. 2012), but the measurements produced provide no information on the speciation of the released material. The detection of particle releases has also advanced, but gathering information on the compositions of those particles within the matrix into which they have been released remains challenging. Both the strong elemental signals from the matrix and the presence of naturally occurring nanoparticles complicate the analyses.

Some progress has been made in assessing both particle release and composition. For example, single-walled CNTs can be separated from soil and sediment and quantified with near-infrared fluorescence spectroscopy (Schierz et al. 2012). C_{60} and C_{70} fullerenes have been extracted from soils using ultrasound and quantified by HPLC-MS (Perez et al. 2013), and from urine (Benn et al. 2011). Single-particle ICP-MS methods have been developed that have proved useful for metal nanoparticles, such as gold and silver (Heithmar 2011; Mitrano et al. 2012) in pore water extracted from soil. Those are examples of methods that rely on separation of nanomaterials from or within a matrix followed by analysis, but concern that the separation process itself can transform the materials remains (von der Kammer et al. 2012). Separation methods that lack stationary phases, such as field-flow fractionation, show the most promise for separating nanomaterials without altering them (Mitrano et al. 2012). Other approaches to monitoring environmental transformations that obviate separation include monitoring of the transformation of tethered nanoparticles (Glover et al. 2011) and use of x-ray–based spectroscopic methods that provide speciation information in media without the need to desiccate samples (Lawrence et al. 2012; Lombi et al. 2012; Lowry et al. 2012b). The generality of the new approaches and their relevance to real-world samples remain to be determined.

There has been some progress toward this objective, but proper characterization of nanomaterial releases will require additional progress in developing methods that can simultaneously determine the particulate characteristics and the nanomaterial composition (including surface chemistry) of the released material. Thus, the committee's assessment is that progress toward this goal should be graded as yellow.

- *Modeling nanomaterial releases along the value chain*

Models are needed for accurate prediction of nanomaterial releases, environmental concentrations, and human and ecosystem exposures. Models of releases also are needed to identify the form and speciation of released nanomaterials. To date, modeling efforts appear to be confined to specific release points and routes of exposure (such as inhalation exposure in the workplace and releases in wastewater-treatment plant effluent discharges). Further progress has not been initiated, because of the lack of information on inventories in the value chains highlighted above. Because of the lack of quantitative information throughout the life cycle of ENMs on which to build such models, progress in this indicator is denoted as red.

Processes That Affect Both Exposure and Hazard

In its first report, the committee highlighted the need to identify the critical nanomaterial interactions that affect ENM behaviors. It recommended identifying cross-cutting processes (for example, agglomeration, aggregation, dissolution, and deposition) that are common to assessing exposure and assessing hazard. Identifying nanomaterial interactions requires cataloging the types of ENM transformations in complex matrices and the time scales associated with the transformations, developing instrumentation to monitor transformations in vivo or in complex environmental media, and developing models to predict ENM behaviors. Integral to these efforts are the need to develop the ontology to describe "transformed" nanomaterials and the need to develop the infrastructure to archive data that enables model development and identification of these processes. Progress ranged from yellow for initiation of basic studies that are beginning to characterize likely types of ENM transformations and to require additional study and for studies that begin to relate ENM properties to observed effects in more complex systems to red for development of new instrumentation to measure transformations in situ, in vivo, or on single particles. The committee also notes that the data generated have not been effectively used to develop and validate the models, because of the absence of a central structured database for consistent documentation of research results.

- *Steps taken toward development of a knowledge infrastructure able to describe the diversity and dynamics of nanomaterials and their transformations in complex biologic and environmental media*

In its first report, the committee indicated the need to develop a knowledge infrastructure to measure and describe nanomaterial behaviors, including transformations that affect exposure and hazard. The types and nature of the transformations that affect both exposure and toxicity studies (for example, aggregation,

Assessment of Progress

agglomeration, oxidation, reduction, dissolution, adsorption of macromolecules, and interactions of ENMs with cell membranes) have been documented in many studies and review articles (Verma and Stellacci 2009; Wiesner et al. 2009; Levard et al. 2012; Lowry et al. 2012a; Moghadam et al. 2012; Mu et al. 2012; Nowack et al. 2012; Cheng et al. 2013; Zhu et al. 2013). The importance of the components of the media in which ENMs are dispersed is also well established (Maiorano et al. 2010). Despite a large volume of laboratory-based research, the committee classifies progress as yellow because no knowledge base exists to describe and understand these transformations in general. Most studies have examined specific conditions, so current understanding of ENM behaviors is system-specific. Knowledge of the mechanisms behind the transformations is also often incomplete. Several nascent efforts are under way to characterize systematically and precisely how various solution conditions (for example, dissolved solutes, pH, and redox state) and ENM properties affect transformations that will allow the development of predictive models (Ottofuelling et al. 2011; Nel et al. 2013). However, the data infrastructure needed to share the results is not yet widely available, as highlighted above. Development of the infrastructure and data-sharing are complicated by the highly variable nature of the transformations and by the lack of an ontology to describe the "state" of a fully or partially transformed ENM. Finally, there is no way to characterize many of the transformations in relevant media at realistic concentrations. In some cases, that will require the development of new instrumentation, as described below. The lack of an ontology and a mechanism for data synthesis led to categorizing this indicator as yellow.

Progress in developing instrumentation to measure key nanomaterial properties and changes in them in complex biologic and environmental media

Measurement of nanomaterial transformations in relevant biologic and environmental media has high priority. In those complex media, a wide array of substantial or subtle changes involving material composition and structure may occur. Adsorption of natural organic matter, proteins, and lipids may change the surface coating. Etching, degradation, or agglomeration of nanoparticle cores may transform the material. Oxidation and dissolution or sulfidation may occur (Liu et al. 2012). Measurements of the materials are further complicated by their presence at low concentrations and in a wide variety of compartments.

Little progress has been made in this indicator despite its importance and the recognition that such measurements are crucial for accelerating nanotechnology EHS research. Several sections in this chapter describe how analytic techniques are being adapted and used in combination to gain information about the composition and structure of ENMs in simple well-characterized media. This indicator is focused on the development of new instrumentation that can measure core and surface compositions and physical dimensions in complex biologic or environmental matrices and in some cases at a single particle resolution. The optimal methods would permit measurement of size and composition in the matrices. Some publications have called for improved detectors to enable single-particle ICP-MS and to improve the spatial resolution of x-ray microprobes (von der Kammer et al. 2012).

Instruments for measuring airborne ENMs are being developed. J. Wang et al. (2011) have developed a universal nanoparticle analyzer to measure and characterize airborne nanoparticle agglomerates. Rhoads et al. (2003) designed an instrument (rapid single-particle mass spectrometry, RSMS-11) to analyze the chemical composition of airborne nanoparticles (less than 20-nm), and efforts are directed at developing an instrument to measure nanoparticle-bound reactive oxygen species in real time (Y. Wang et al. 2011). Despite those developments, overall progress is insufficient.

Considerable progress is required to meet current and future needs in the nanotechnology-EHS field, and little headway has been made toward the necessary instrumentation. Therefore, this objective is labeled red by the committee.

Initiation of interdisciplinary research that can relate native nanomaterial structures to transformations that occur in organisms and as a result of biologic processes

In its first report, the committee emphasized the importance of processes that lead to transformations of ENMs in organisms or ecosystems. Adsorption of proteins, lipids, and organic materials may alter surface properties of ENMs, form a corona, affect mechanisms of cell interactions, and alter ENM biokinetics. (The corona, a coating that binds to the surface of ENMs, influences the biodistribution and effects of ENMs [Walczyk et al. 2010].) Although the concept of "differential adsorption" of lipids and proteins has been described (Müller and Heinemann 1989) and has been developed in vitro (Cedervall et al. 2007; Walcyzk et al. 2010), the committee identified a major gap in understanding of the effects, particularly in vivo effects, of the types and amounts of adsorbed lipids and proteins.

Some progress has been made by several laboratories in the United States and Europe that are investigating the adsorption of lipids and proteins on ENMs introduced into organisms or when interacting with biologic media in vitro. Although in vitro studies have advanced this field of research considerably (for example, showing that modifying ENM surfaces by coating them with proteins or surfactants can result in altered cellular responses), confirmatory in vivo studies are lacking. Despite the progress, much research is needed. The importance of other ENM transformations (altered surfaces, agglomeration, deagglomeration, aggregation, and solubilization) for biokinetics and effects needs to be considered. In addition, studies have focused on acute short-term effects, and little is known about the persistence of such effects in vivo. Moreover, effects of chronic low-dose exposure are not well established. Phenomena observed at high doses may not be entirely relevant in vivo inasmuch as dose may influence mechanisms (Slikker et al. 2004).

Assessment of Progress 61

Formulation of time-course studies will be essential for in vivo and in vitro evaluations. They are necessary for documenting the possible transformations of ENM characteristics within the life cycle and for assessing the persistence of measured responses in organisms. The latter issue will be essential for identifying and characterizing hazards. The mixed progress in these subjects led the committee to assess this indicator as yellow.

- *Extent of use of experimental research results in initial models for predicting nanomaterial behavior in complex biologic and environmental settings*

The fate and effects of ENMs in complex environments will be determined by a set of interactions between the materials and the properties of the environments. Identifying mechanisms by which those interactions occur requires integration of the mechanistic understanding gained from studies on a laboratory scale in well-controlled environments and the understanding obtained from research conducted in environments of varied complexity. Predictive models can then be developed on the basis of the mechanisms identified in relevant exposure scenarios. In contrast with the development of models for specific behaviors (such as aggregation and agglomeration) in relatively well-characterized environments, development of models for predicting nanomaterial behavior in complex biologic and environmental systems has seen little progress. One key limitation is the lack of resources for conducting long-term experiments in large-scale environmental systems, such as mesocosms[6], or for performing in vivo studies. Another is the absence of a central structured database for consistent documentation of research results that permits datasets to be compared and used in models. Some efforts are under way in EPA–NSF funded centers to develop models for predicting nanomaterial behavior in complex biologic and environmental systems, but they are disjointed. Data collected in the various systems (environments and organisms) are not characterized in the same manner and are therefore not readily usable for modeling. In addition, the focus has been on only a few ENMs, so comparisons among ENMs that have different chemical composition are not possible. The committee therefore identified this indicator as red.

Nanomaterial Interactions in Complex Systems Ranging from Subcellular Systems to Ecosystems

In its first report, the committee recognized the need to investigate and increase the understanding of interactions of ENMs in a variety of complex systems. Complex systems can range from subcellular organelles to cells to organisms to ecosystems. These elements may act independently, synergistically, or antagonistically in response to ENM exposures. Research efforts that focus on system-level approaches to investigate potential ENM effects on human health

---

[6]A means of studying the natural environment under controlled conditions.

and the environment are needed. Indirect effects may also result from direct interactions with ENMs. For example, ENM transformations that occur in environmental systems—for example, through weathering in ecosystems or metabolism in organisms and ecosystems—may have unexpected effects on other organisms along the food chain or indirectly in organ systems. Specifically quantum dots have been found to be toxic to a variety of systems, but weathering of quantum dots can induce antibiotic resistance in some bacterial strains that could in turn affect organisms that are susceptible to these bacteria (Yang et al. 2012). In mammals, inhaled ENMs that are deposited in the distal lung or alveolar epithelial sites may interact with lung lining fluids to form nanomaterial–corona complexes that may alter the disposition and biologic activity of the ENM. Therefore, a first step is to identify relevant exposure sources, concentrations, and cellular and ecologic targets so that potential effects on complex systems can be addressed. Research progress indicators for this category ranged from yellow to red; no indicators were denoted as green. Indicators were yellow for extent of initiation of studies that address effects of ENMs in complex systems, adaptation of system-level tools to support studies in these systems, and steps toward development of models for assessing ecologic exposures and effects. Indicators were red for developing screening tools that reflect important toxicity pathways and identifying benchmark and reference ENMs for use in studies to estimate exposure or dose.

- *Extent of initiation of studies that address the impacts of nanomaterials on a variety of end points in complex systems, such as studies that link in vitro to in vivo observations, that examine effects on important biologic pathways, and that investigate ecosystem effects*[7]

The majority of toxicology studies involving ENMs have examined only a few end points, including acute mortality and acute oxidative stress. Although valuable, these studies provide little information that is useful for examining the effects of ENM exposures on organisms. Historical studies of chemicals have demonstrated that evaluation of outcomes—such as reproductive, developmental, and endocrine effects—is critical for understanding human health and ecologic impacts. In vitro analyses, although potentially useful as an initial screen for gross effects, have not been shown to predict in vivo effects adequately. Ecosystem effects, which are difficult to measure, are often not considered in chemical assessments, but such information is essential for understanding changes in community and abiotic interactions that may lead to detrimental effects. Initial model ecosystem studies on mescocosms can begin to address changes that may occur on a larger scale due to ENM releases. In addition, mo-

---

[7]This indicator was formerly titled "Extent of initiation of studies that address heretofore underrepresented fields of research, such as those seeking to relate in vitro to in vivo observations, to predict ecosystem effects, or to examine effects on the endocrine or developmental systems" in NRC (2012, p. 182).

lecular studies can provide the basis to predict potential larger scale impacts. Conduct of these more complex studies, rather than reliance on data from more simplified assays, is critical for comprehensive understanding of the potential effects of ENMs on humans and ecosystems.

Nanotoxicology studies to determine the suitability of in vitro study results for predicting responses in vivo had been published before the release of the committee's first report (Sayes et al. 2007; Gerde 2008; Lu et al. 2009; Rushton et al. 2010; Han et al. 2012; Zhang et al. 2012), but the report identified several subjects that required further in-depth study. Continuing concerns include dosimetry-related issues and the need for further in vivo validation of effects and underlying mechanisms. The committee also identified a dearth of exposure-assessment studies—that is, studies of workplace exposures and consumer exposures to ENMs.

Some studies have addressed the latter subject, including workplace-exposure studies and ecosystem studies that were conducted by EPA–NSF funded centers. NIOSH and academic institutions (Bello et al. 2009; Methner et al. 2010; NIOSH 2012a; Tsai et al. 2012) have increased efforts to engage with industry to perform workplace monitoring. The European NanoCare Program also includes exposure-assessment studies (Kuhlbusch et al. 2011).

With respect to in vitro–in vivo correlations, several studies have compared results of in vitro and in vivo toxicity testing for their predictive power. The comparisons have provided findings that encompass good and poor concordance between in vitro and in vivo results (for example, Sayes et al. 2007; Rushton et al. 2010); this indicates a need for improved approaches to the design of comparative studies with the goal of predicting hazards. High-throughput screening (HTS) assays allow hazard ranking of many ENMs simultaneously on the basis of mechanistic information about cellular activation pathways of injury (Meng et al. 2009). However, Thomas et al. (2012a, b) concluded from an evaluation of HTS assays of numerous chemicals that these assays have little ability to predict in vivo hazards. They can, however, be useful for setting priorities among materials for further testing (Dix et al. 2012).

Validation of the predictive value of HTS assays for assessing in vivo hazards of ENMs is essential, including consideration of and differences between short-term, intermediate, and chronic exposures. Study designs should focus on developing tests with relevant ENM dosimetry and realistic doses (based on exposure data) and on time-course assessment to gauge the persistence of measured end points. The cell types used should simulate in vivo point-of-entry exposure routes. Selection of relevant doses for cell types of secondary organs should be based on results of biokinetic studies. In the aggregate, those integrated components are necessary for developing science-based in vivo predictability and extrapolation. With regard to acute-hazard ranking, HTS assays can be powerful, but present approaches for short-term and long-term hazard assessments and corresponding risk characterization have serious limitations. Furthermore, only a few long-term in vivo studies have examined more sensitive end points, such as reproduction and growth, and few funded studies other than those supported through EPA–NSF funded centers have examined ecosystem effects.

Some other subjects that remain underrepresented are toxicity mechanisms and pathways examined under realistic exposure conditions, exposure to mixtures of contaminants, genotoxicity, and ecosystem effects of ENM exposures. Therefore, the committee designates progress in these fields as yellow.

- *Extent of adaptation of existing system-level tools (such as individual species tests, microcosms, and organ-system models) to support studies of nanomaterials in such systems*

In its first report, the committee noted inadequate activity in this indicator. Specific studies would contribute to a better understanding of system-level effects that can be induced by ENMs in an organism or in the environment. Adaptation of existing system-level tools to support studies of isolated organ systems—isolated perfused heart or lung, explant models (isolated vessels, including coronary vessels and aorta, and muscle), in vitro double- and triple-cell models, and complete constructs of airway epithelium—have been developed and used in nanotoxicologic research, either through exposure of live organisms to ENMs or through exposure of the isolated model systems directly (Nurkiewicz et al. 2008). Such models are useful for exploring mechanisms of specific effects, preferably if appropriate doses have been selected for exposure of the organism or the explant.

Whole-organism environmental studies have been adapted to be used in nanotoxicology (Lovern and Klaper 2006; Bai et al. 2010; Galloway et al. 2010; H. Wang et al. 2009; S. Wang et al. 2011). Specific projects that are addressing systemwide effects of ENM exposures include studies of the use of microcosms and mesocosms to examine organism and ecosystem-level effects (Priester et al. 2012; Colman et al. 2013). Those studies demonstrate that steps toward meeting this objective have been initiated, but progress is confined to a few studies, and system-level effects remain largely unknown. The committee therefore determined that this indicator is yellow.

- *Development of a set of screening tools that reflect important characteristics or toxicity pathways of the complex systems described above*[8]

As noted in the committee's first report, hazard-identification studies of a variety of ENMs have used both in vivo and in vitro methods. Development of a set of reliable and validated screening tools is critical in that adequate testing of individual ENMs used in commerce, each with different functionalities and ap-

---

[8]This indicator was originally phrased as "Extent of refinement of a set of screening tools that reflect important characteristics or toxicity pathways of the complex systems described above" (NRC 2012, p. 182).

plications, is not practical. In general, results obtained from in vivo studies may have limited value for assessing health risks due to use of higher doses of ENMs than might be expected from real-world exposures and a focus primarily on acute responses. However, implementation of a spectrum of in vitro investigations may ultimately hold promise for revealing important mechanistic insights into toxicity pathways. Optimizing the relevance of in vitro studies to toxicity considerations would require experimental designs that involve dose–response behavior over a full range of doses (very low to high) in relevant cell types, including time-course assessments and validation of findings with corresponding in vivo systems.

Chapter 3 of the first report, "Critical Questions for Understanding Human and Environmental Effects of Engineered Nanomaterials", posed the question (p. 91), What biologic effects occur at realistic ENM doses and dose rates, and how do ENM properties influence the magnitude of these effects? The report noted that a long-term goal is to develop simple in vitro assays that predict in vivo effects at the organism level and may eventually be used for HTS assays. To address that long-term goal, it was concluded that a key requirement should be that any in vitro assay used as a predictive tool needs to have been validated with appropriate and pertinent in vivo data (with particular relevance to exposure routes). The results of simple assays have been proposed for identifying potential effects and possibly establishing a hazard scale (Rushton et al. 2010), although some comparative studies have reported a lack of convergence between in vivo–related (inhalation or intratracheal instillation) findings and in vitro data on the same nanoparticle test materials, perhaps partly because of mechanisms that are dose-dependent (Slikker et al. 2004; Sayes et al. 2007, 2009; Warheit et al. 2009) or because of differential ENM transformations that depend on the exposure vehicle (medium) used (Lowry et al. 2012a). Finally, as currently designed, in vitro studies are limited by their inherent measurement of acute responses. Even if they are conducted under relevant dose conditions, in vitro results generally reflect early (acute) effects of exposures and may not predict long-term (chronic) effects.

Research activity to correlate in vivo mechanistic toxicity studies systematically at relevant concentrations with in vitro screening assays that use relevant exposure concentrations, ENMs, cell types, and appropriate routes of exposures (such as inhalation, oral, dermal, and intravenous exposure) is central to progress. Some initial efforts have been proposed to address that issue in the ToxCast and NIEHS U19[9] programs. Laboratories are pursuing such research, and important insights into mechanisms of toxicity are being generated, but these efforts are not sufficient to provide the information necessary for adequate un-

---

[9]U19 is part the National Institute of Environmental Health Sciences Centers for Nanotechnology Health Implications Research. It is an interdisciplinary program that comprises five U19 and three cooperative centers and other grantees and is intended to increase understanding of how the properties of ENMs influence their interactions with biologic systems and potential health risks.

derstanding of toxicity pathways in cell and organ systems. The committee designates this indicator as red given the limited progress in appropriately designed studies.

- *Steps toward development of models for exposure and potential ecologic effects*[10]

Work on modeling exposure to and effects of nanomaterials in ecosystems, including food webs, is in its infancy. Important first steps have been taken to understand the phenomena of uptake, bioaccumulation, and trophic transfer (Werlin et al. 2011; Unrine et al. 2012), and this mixed progress gives this indicator a yellow rating.

However, more work is required to understand the mechanisms of biouptake. Lack of progress in modeling the transfer of materials between organisms can be attributed in part to the relatively low priority that this topic has received, as measured by publications, relative to work on direct health effects (see Figure 3-3 in NRC 2012). In addition, the modeling required is predicated on fundamental discovery concerning the mechanisms of biouptake and assimilation of ENMs in organisms. Greater focus on modeling of biouptake, bioaccumulation, and trophic transfer is essential not only for predicting the fate of nanomaterials in ecosystems but for interpreting the growing body of literature on nanomaterial effects associated with ambient concentrations introduced in laboratory studies. In addition to uptake, more information is needed on the effects of chronic, low-level realistic exposure scenarios in complex ecologic systems. Effects of ENMs in a simplified assay may not accurately reflect the gross effects on a system of interconnected species. Alterations in uptake in the presence of multiple species, population and community effects, changes in interactions among organisms, transformation of ENMs, and such changes in abiotic factors as nutrients because of nanomaterials are all important variables that need more research attention.

- *Identification of benchmark (positive and negative) and reference materials*[11] *for use in studies and measurement tools and methods to estimate exposure and dose in complex systems.*

---

[10]The indicator originally titled "Steps toward development of models for exposure and potential effects along the ecologic food chain" (NRC 2012, p. 182) was rephrased to broaden its scope to include all ecologic effects (both biotic and abiotic).

[11]The committee differentiates between benchmark materials and reference materials. Reference Material, defined by ISO (2006), is a "material, sufficiently homogenous and stable with respect to one or more specified properties, which has been established to be fit for its intended use in a measurement process". The focus is on its physicochemical properties and its use in metrology when certified by national or international agencies (for example, NIST gold nanoparticles and TiO_2 nanoparticles). Benchmark materials are well-characterized physicochemically and toxicologically, and can serve as positive or

The committee's first report identified a pressing need to establish reference materials for all aspects of nanomaterial-related research. Availability of toxicity benchmark materials (positive and negative) and reference materials for metrology are of high value for hazard ranking and risk assessment. NIST has issued two well-characterized, certified reference nanomaterials, TiO_2 (P-25[12]) and gold (10, 30, and 60 nm), that could be used in toxicologic studies.

The International Organization for Standardization defines a reference material as a "material, sufficiently homogeneous and stable with respect to one or more specified properties, which has been established to be fit for its intended use in a measurement process" (ISO 2006). Therefore, existing reference materials are standards solely for material characterization (for example, NIST gold nanoparticles, standard reference material RM 8011, 8012, and 8013) or for standardizing measurement instrumentation. Benchmark materials for use in toxicologic and ecotoxicologic research need to be carefully characterized with respect to both physicochemical and toxicologic properties. The latter probably depend on several physicochemical properties (for example ENM size, charge, or in vivo solubility) that may make it necessary to establish more than one reference material for hazard ranking. Generally accepted positive or negative benchmark materials for toxicologic purposes have not yet been identified, but suggestions have been made in some individual studies (Aitken et al. 2008; Stone et al. 2010). Well-characterized benchmark ENMs should serve as references against which new and untested ENMs can be ranked as an initial step in hazard identification. Such information, with exposure data, can serve as a basis of risk assessment. The committee therefore believes that overall progress in this objective is inadequate and therefore has designated it red.

INDICATORS OF PROGRESS IN IMPLEMENTATION

Enhancing Interagency Coordination

In its first report, the committee acknowledged the value of the coordinating role played by the NNI and pointed to some changes that have enhanced interagency coordination, including the naming of an NNCO EHS coordinator by the Office of Science and Technology Policy (OSTP). However, the committee concluded in its first report (p. 169) and continues to believe that accountability for implementation of the NNI EHS research strategy is limited and hampered by the absence of an entity that has sufficient management and budgetary authority to direct implementation throughout NNI agencies and to ensure its integration with EHS research being undertaken in the private sector, the academic community, and international organizations. Ensuring implementation of

---

negative controls for comparing exposure-dose-response relationships of nanomaterials in toxicologic tests and in risk assessment.

[12]P-25 is the product number for titanium dioxide.

the strategy and gauging progress in high-priority research also requires an assessment of the effectiveness of available mechanisms for interagency collaboration and frequent periodic identification—not just of recent, current, or newly initiated interagency research collaborations but also of funding needs. The committee's assessment of progress against its two indicators for interagency collaboration is as follows.

Progress toward establishing a mechanism to ensure sufficient management and budgetary authority to develop and implement an EHS research strategy among NNI agencies

The committee reviewed the NNI's 2011 research strategy and its 2013 budget supplement, which show considerable progress in coordination among NNI agencies on EHS research. Favorable developments include the addition of FDA and CPSC research programs to the NNI's EHS budget "crosscut", an increased focus by the Nanotechnology Environmental Health Implications working group on identifying opportunities for cross-agency collaborations, joint solicitations and funding of research by multiple NNI agencies, and clearer tracking of research against the NNI's broad goals and designated program component areas. The NNI strategy and budget documents also identify numerous plans to foster additional interagency collaboration, although the extent to which the plans have been or are being implemented appears to be limited on the basis of input received by the committee at its November 2012 workshop and discussions with NNCO staff.

However, as highlighted in the committee's first report, the need extends well beyond better coordination among NNI agencies, a role that the NNCO is fulfilling. Therefore, the committee identified as an indicator of progress the establishment of a mechanism that would have sufficient management and budgetary authority to ensure implementation of the NNI's EHS research strategy. The committee has not discerned substantial progress on this indicator, so it is marked red.

The committee is not alone in raising the need for a more centralized and accountable authority. In its fourth assessment of the NNI, the President's Council of Advisors on Science and Technology (PCAST 2012) noted the "lack of integration between nanotechnology-related EHS research . . . and the kind of information policymakers need to effectively manage potential risks from nanomaterials" (p. vi); it called on the NNI to establish "high-level, cross-agency authoritative and accountable governance" (p. viii) even as it acknowledged changes made to enhance coordination of research efforts among NNI agencies. Similarly, a recent Government Accountability Office report (GAO 2012) that reviewed the NNI's research strategy and associated activities identified substantial instances of interagency research collaborations[13] but also the absence of "outcome-related performance measures, targets or time frames that allow for monitoring and reporting on progress toward meeting the research needs" (p. 46).

The 2012 PCAST review of the NNI made several specific recommendations for OSTP to strengthen the NNCO "to broaden its impact and efficacy and improve its ability to coordinate *and develop* NNI programs and policies related to those programs" (p. 19; italics added). With respect to program management, the review noted that "PCAST is concerned that the agency representatives appointed to the NSET Subcommittee do not have a level of authority within their agencies to influence budget allocations needed to meet NNI objectives" (p. vi), reiterating the 2010 PCAST recommendation that OSTP "require each agency in the NNI to have senior representatives with decision-making authority participate in coordination activities of the NNI" (p. 39). The NNI's response to the 2010 recommendation is included in its 2013 budget supplement (NSET 2012a) under the heading "Recommendations considered but actions unlikely or not needed" (p. 61); this indicates that the NNI considers its current structure to be sufficient and intends to maintain it.

The committee remains concerned about the absence of a clear, central convening authority in the NNI structure and considers it a serious gap in the NNI's ability to implement an effective EHS research strategy.

- *Extent to which the NNCO is annually identifying funding needs for interagency collaboration on critical high-priority research*

The NNI and its member agencies have made considerable progress toward increased collaboration in EHS research, including issuance of its 2011 EHS research strategy. As noted above, the committee's review of the NNI's strategy and the NNI's 2013 budget supplement identified numerous examples of current and planned cross-agency collaborations. The examples demonstrate that multiple NNI agencies are and plan to continue jointly conducting intramural research and jointly sponsor and fund solicitations for extramural research. The NNI has also instituted a clearer means of tracking in its budget supplement how current research aligns with its broad goals and new strategy. However, concerns have been raised by committee members that jointly funded research is not being managed jointly and that joint research solicitations have been relatively open-ended and not sufficiently strategically aligned to key research needs. The NNI's signature initiatives (NNI 2012) offer another potential means of fostering collaboration in EHS research; although focused now only on nanotechnology development, they encompass such efforts as the multiagency Nano-

---

[13] A helpful list of collaborative agreements between NNI agencies is provided as Appendix II of the GAO report. It is notable, however, that many of the agreements date back several years, and none is listed as having been initiated in 2012; this suggests that momentum in the activity may have waned recently.

technology Knowledge Infrastructure and the Nanoinformatics 2020 Roadmap, both of which are aimed at developing the infrastructure needed to collect, analyze, and share nanotechnology-related information (NSET 2012b)—which could readily be extended to include EHS-related information.

The committee continues to believe that accountability for fostering interagency collaboration in implementing the strategy requires not only identifying what collaborative research is under way or contemplated, but having in place a rigorous means of estimating periodically (ideally at least annually) the levels and sources of funding needed to ensure that interagency research efforts have sufficient funding to meet specific goals and complete high-priority research. That need echoes the calls by PCAST (2010, 2012) and GAO (2012) for the NNI to develop and implement better performance metrics that can be used to track progress against core objectives. The committee's progress indicator focuses on identifying funding needs for collaborative efforts between agencies to accelerate and enhance progress in high-priority research. The committee has not been made aware of any effort by the NNCO to develop such a mechanism and renews its call for the NNCO to do so. Because of the limited progress made in addressing this indicator, the committee denotes it yellow.

Providing for Stakeholder Engagement in the Research Strategy

Progress toward actively engaging diverse stakeholders in a continuing manner in all aspects of strategy development, implementation, and revision

This indicator represents a very high but achievable bar for stakeholder engagement, seeking broad engagement both in a continuing manner and in all aspects of the strategy. It seems clear that this high bar has not been cleared although the committee notes examples of progress. The stakeholder community includes government and academic researchers, nongovernment organizations, regulators, industry, nanotechnology workers, and of course consumers. The committee's workshop sought to hear from representatives of each of those communities and did so successfully. Representatives of the various groups were well informed of the process and need but also frustrated by the lack of pull from the NNI EHS community for their involvement. Certainly, none could point to a recurring and inclusive forum for their involvement and participation.

The committee, however, notes several examples of progress toward the goals. The committee workshop was one such example. Another, more prominent case is the NIOSH-sponsored Safe Nano by Design Conference, which took place in Albany, NY, in August 2012 (NIOSH 2012b) that was specifically focused on NIOSH priorities. The creation and recurrence of similar forums that engage the range of EHS stakeholders would be a positive step. This indicator is yellow given that some progress has been observed. However, further engagement through such forums on all other aspects of strategy development, imple-

Conducting and Communicating the Results of Research Funded Through Public–Private Partnerships

Progress toward establishment of effective public–private partnerships, as measured by such steps as completion of partnership agreements, issuance of requests for proposal, and establishment of a sound governance structure

In its first report, the committee identified the need for public–private partnerships (PPPs) to help to implement the four broad, high-priority research categories of its research strategy. The need for PPPs is driven by the need to supplement and leverage federal funding and by the importance of having private stakeholders (such as manufacturers) actively involved in the research. For example, data on reference materials, nanomaterial product inventories, and the release of nanomaterials through the value chain are critical inputs into the research; one good way to provide such information accurately is to establish formal partnerships between government agencies, manufacturers, and other key stakeholders—such as academe—that are involved in implementing the research strategy.

Progress in creating well-defined, effective partnerships as measured by partnership agreements, issuance of requests for proposals, and the establishment of governance structure is poor, so this indicator is red. NIOSH provides the closest examples. A summary report by NIOSH (2012a) covering the period 2004–2011 describes accomplishments and research findings from surveys in a research and development laboratory, in commercial nanoscale metal oxide production facilities, in a facility engaged in development of optical products with quantum dot coatings, and in a facility that spins nylon nanofibers. Other surveys included MWCNT manufacturers, metal oxide manufacturers, nano-enhanced silica iron absorbent manufacturers and additional diverse nanoscale-material producing laboratories. Those surveys do not represent formal PPPs, but they were performed on the basis of a NIOSH–manufacturer collaborative effort by conducting over 40 field assessments in nanomaterial manufacturer and user facilities. In another example, the Nanoparticle Occupational Safety and Health consortium—comprising 16 members in industry (for example, Procter and Gamble and DuPont), federal agencies (for example, NIOSH), and nonprofit organizations (Environmental Defense Fund)—tackled issues of the measurement of nanoparticles and the efficiency of filtration materials for engineered nanoparticles, evaluation of bioactivity of silicon nanowires in the consortium's partnership with IBM, and understanding of and improvement in exposure controls for fullerenes and other engineered nanoparticles in its partnership with Luna Nano (NOSH 2007).

Overall, the main impediments to creating PPPs are the lack of agreement on needed elements of a governance structure, disparate core objectives between public and private entities, insufficient funding commitments from both government and industry, and confidentiality concerns. In Chapter 4, the committee provides recommendations and examples of best practices to alleviate those road blocks.

Managing Potential Conflicts of Interest

In its first report, the committee noted that the NNI's dual functions—developing and promoting nanotechnology and its applications and mitigating risks arising from such applications—pose tensions or even actual conflicts between its goals. Manifestations of the tension previously noted by the committee included the vastly disparate allocation of resources between the two functions, the inadequacy of EHS risk research funding, and the NNI's classification of research projects with respect to their "EHS relevance". The committee believes that the tension can also affect the extramural research community, especially EHS risk researchers in large centers, the bulk of whose research funding is focused on applications. To address what it saw as an inherent conflict, the committee concluded that a clear separation in the management and budgetary authority and accountability between the functions was needed, and it identified two indicators for tracking progress in managing conflicts of interest. That conclusion echoed that of a previous National Research Council report (2009), which noted that "a clear separation of accountability for development of applications and assessment of potential implication of nanotechnology would help ensure that the public health implications has appropriate priority" (NRC 2009, p. 11).

Progress toward achieving a clear separation in management and budgetary authority and accountability between the functions of developing and promoting applications of nanotechnology and understanding and assessing its potential health and environmental implications

The committee sees little progress in establishing clear and discernibly separate management and budgetary structure between the two potentially conflicting functions in the NNI itself or the agencies that pursue or fund research on both applications and EHS risk implications of engineered nanomaterials. Therefore, this indicator is red. Both functions continue to operate under the same management and budget structures in the NNI and in its member agencies. In its first report, the committee noted possible models and mechanisms that could be used to separate accountability for the NNI's dual functions, for example, elevating oversight of the EHS research portfolio in OSTP (NRC 2012; pp. 166–169), assigning responsibility and comparable authority for the two functions to different offices or to senior staff members in individual agencies or in the NNI itself (NRC 2012; pp.167, 173–174), or separating the two functions into independent entities—a model used elsewhere to address potentially conflicting issues related to nuclear power (p. 174). The committee acknowledges that in the absence of a change in its statutory mandate, the NNI would be hard-pressed to establish wholly separate management and budgetary structures and authorities for its dual functions. In the absence of such a change, the committee encourages the NNI and participating agencies to consider other approaches for managing perceived or actual conflicts of interest and biases. If not adequately addressed, such perceptions could undermine public trust and confidence in the research, technology, and government processes that are meant to ensure the health, and safety of ENMs.

Continued separate tracking and reporting of EHS research activities and funding distinct from those for other, more basic or application-oriented research

The NNI has made considerable progress on this issue, commencing before the committee issued its first report. That progress constitutes an impressive step toward creating the transparency noted above. The Office of Management and Budget (OMB) call to NNI agencies for detailed information on FY 2009 EHS research project funding facilitated easier identification of research projects most directly relevant to EHS risk. That data call helped to inform the NNI's Environmental, Health, and Safety Research Strategy (NSET 2011). The NNI supplement to the president's 2013 budget (NSET 2012a) also provides narrative information on agency-specific EHS research activities and projects.

Despite the impressive progress, the tracking of EHS research progress and performance between and within NNI agencies remains challenging. As noted by GAO in its May 2012 report, performance information— such as outcomes, outputs, quality, timeliness, customer satisfaction, and efficiency—can inform such critical management decisions as priority-setting and resource allocation. Without project-specific information, researchers and other stakeholders have only a vague understanding of the research questions, methods, materials, and study populations being addressed through the NNI. Although periodic OMB data calls for EHS research project funding are helpful and could be made even more helpful if they included clearer guidance on how agencies should differentiate research directly relevant to EHS risk from applications research with EHS implications, they cannot address the need for a continuing (ideally annual) system for identifying and tracking EHS research projects and their performance.

REFERENCES

Aitken, R.J., S.M. Hankin, C.L. Tran, K. Donaldson, V. Stone, P. Cumpson, J. Johnstone, Q. Chaudhry, S. Cash, and J. Garrod. 2008. A multidisciplinary approach to the identification of reference materials for engineered nanoparticle toxicology. Nantoxicology 2(2):71-78.

AZoNano.com. 2010. Nanotechnology Characterization Laboratory Partners with NIEHS for Physicochemical Characterization of Engineered Nanomaterials. News: November 12, 2010 [online]. Available: http://www.azonano.com/news.aspx?news ID=20509 [accessed Jan. 24, 2013].

Bai, W., Z. Zhang, W. Tian, X. He, Y. Ma, Y. Zhao, and Z. Chai. 2010. Toxicity of zinc oxide nanoparticles to zebrafish embryo: A physicochemical study of toxicity mechanism. J. Nanopart. Res. 12(5):1645-1654.

Bello, D., B.L. Wardle, N. Yamamoto, R.G. de Villoria, E.J. Garcia, A.J. Hart, K. Ahn, M.J. Ellenbecker, and M. Hallock. 2009. Exposure to nanoscale particles and fibers during machining of hybrid advanced composites containing nanotubes. J. Nanopart. Res. 11(1):231-249.

Benn, T.M., B.F. Pycke, P. Herckes, P. Westerhoff, and R.U. Halden. 2011. Evaluation of extraction methods for quantification of aqueous fullerenes in urine. Anal. Bioanal. Chem. 399(4):1631-1639.

Bernhardt, E.S., B.P. Colman, M.F. Hochella, Jr., B.J. Cardinale, R.M. Nisbet, C.J. Richardson, and L. Yin. 2010. An ecological perspective on nanomaterial impacts in the environment. J. Environ. Qual. 39(6):1954-1965.

Bonner, J.C., R.M. Silva, A.J. Taylor, J.M. Brown, S.C. Hilderbrand, V. Castranova, D. Porter, A. Elder, G. Oberdörster, J.R. Harkema, L.A. Bramble, T.J. Kavanagh, D. Botta, A. Nel, and K.E. Pinkerton. 2013. Interlaboratory evaluation of rodent pulmonary responses to engineered nanomaterials: The NIEHS Nano Go Consortium. Environ. Health Perspect. 121(6):676-682.

Cedervall, T., I. Lynch, M. Foy, T. Berggård, S.C. Donnelly, G. Cagney, S. Linse, and K.A. Dawson. 2007. Detailed identification of plasma proteins adsorbed on copolymer nanoparticles. Angew. Chem. Int. 46(30):5754-5756.

Chen, B.T., A. Afshari, S. Stone, M. Jackson, D. Schwegler-Berry, D.G. Frazer, V. Castranova, and T.A. Thomas. 2010. Nanoparticles-containing spray can aerosol: Characterization, exposure assessment, and generator design. Inhal. Toxicol. 22(13):1072-1082.

Cheng, L.C., X.M. Jiang, J. Wang, C.Y. Chen, and R.S. Liu. 2013. Nano-bio effects: Interaction of nanomaterials with cells. Nanoscale 5(9):3547-3569.

Colman, B.P., C.L. Arnaout, S. Anciaux, C.K. Gunsch, M.F. Hochella, Jr., B. Kim, G.V. Lowry, B.M. McGill, B.C. Reinsch, C.J. Richardson, J.M. Unrine, J.P. Wright, L. Yin, and E.S. Bernhardt. 2013. Low concentrations of silver nanoparticles in biosolids cause adverse ecosystem responses under realistic field scenario. PLoS One 8(2):e57189.

Dix, D.J., K.A. Houck, R.S. Judson, N.C. Kleinstreuer, T.B. Knudsen, M.T. Martin, D.M. Reif, A.M. Richard, I. Shah, N.S. Sipes, and R.J. Kavlock. 2012. Incorporating biological, chemical, and toxicological knowledge into predictive models of toxicity. Toxicol. Sci. 130(2):440-441.

EPA (U.S. Environmental Protection Agency). 2012. Increasing Scientific Data on the Fate, Transport and Behavior of Engineered Nanomaterials in Selected Environmental and Biological Matrices. Extramural Research, U.S. Environmental Protection Agency [online]. Available: http://cfpub.epa.gov/ncer_abstracts/index.cfm/fuseaction/recipients.display/rfa_id/534/records_per_page/ALL [accessed Mar. 13, 2013].

Fatisson, J., I.R. Quevedo, K.J. Wilkinson, and N. Tufenkji. 2012. Physicochemical characterization of engineered nanoparticles under physiological conditions: Effect of culture media components and particle surface coating. Colloid Surface B 91:198-204.

Finnish Institute of Occupational Health. 2012. EU-U.S. nanoEHS Community of Research (CORs) Flyer [online]. Available: http://www.ttl.fi/en/international/conferences/senn2012/senn2012_programme/Documents/COR_flyer.pdf [accessed Feb. 1, 2013].

Galloway, T., C. Lewis, I. Dolciotti, B.D. Johnston, J. Moger, and F. Regoli. 2010. Sublethal toxicity of nano-titanium dioxide and carbon nanotubes in a sediment dwelling marine polychaete. Environ. Pollut. 158(5):1748-1755.

GAO (U.S. Government Accountability Office). 2012. Nanotechnology: Improved Performance Information Needed for Environmental, Health, and Safety Research. GAO-12-427. Washington, DC: U.S. Government Accountability Office [online]. Available: http://www.gao.gov/assets/600/591007.pdf [accessed Apr. 4, 2013].

Gerde, P. 2008. How do we compare dose to cells in vitro with dose to live animals and humans? Some experiences with inhaled substances. Exp. Toxicol. Pathol. 60(2-3):181-184.

Glover, R.D., J.M. Miller, and J.E. Hutchison. 2011. Generation of metal nanoparticles from silver and copper objects: Nanoparticle dynamics on surfaces and potential sources of nanoparticles in the environment. ACS Nano 5(11):8950-8957.

Gottschalk, F., and B. Nowack. 2011. The release of engineered nanomaterials to the environment. J. Environ. Monit. 13(5):1145-1155.

Gottschalk, F., C. Ort, R.W. Scholz, and B. Nowack. 2011. Engineered nanomaterials in rivers – Exposure scenarios for Switzerland at high spatial and temporal resolution. Environ. Pollut. 159(12):3439-3445.

Han, X., N. Corson, P. Wade-Mercer, R. Gelein, J. Jiang, M. Sahu, P. Biswas, J.N. Finkelstein, A. Elder, and G. Oberdörster. 2012. Assessing the relevance of in vitro studies in nanotoxicology by examining correlations between in vitro and in vivo data. Toxicology 297(1-3):1-9.

Harper, S.L., J.L. Carriere, J.M. Miller, J.E. Hutchison, B.L.S. Maddux, and R.L. Tanguay. 2011. Systematic evaluation of nanomaterial toxicity: Utility of standardized materials and rapid assays. ACS Nano 5(6):4688-4697.

Helland, A., P. Wick, A. Koehler, K. Schmid, and C. Som. 2007. Reviewing the environmental and human health knowledge base of carbon nanotubes. Environ. Health Perspect. 115(8):1125-1131.

Hendren, C.O., X. Mesnard, J. Droge, and M.R. Wiesner. 2011. Estimating production data for five engineered nanomaterials as a basis for exposure assessment. Environ. Sci. Technol. 45(7):2562-2569.

Heithmar, E.M. 2011. Screening Methods for Metal-Containing Nanoparticles in Water. EPA/600/R-11/096. U.S. Environmental Protection Agency, Washington, DC.

Hou, W.C., P. Westerhoff, and J.D. Posner. 2013. Biological accumulation of engineered nanomaterials: A review of current knowledge. Environ. Sci. Process. Impacts 15(1):103-122.

ILSI (International Life Sciences Institute). 2013a. Nano Release Consumer Products [online]. Available: http://www.ilsi.org/ResearchFoundation/RSIA/Pages/NanoRelease1.aspx [accessed Mar. 29, 2013].

ILSI (International Life Science Institute). 2013b. Nano Character Workshop at NIEHS, January 10-11, 2013, Research Triangle Park, NC [online]. Available: http://www.ilsi.org/NanoCharacter/Pages/2013-Workshop.aspx [accessed Mar. 29, 2013].

ISO (International Organization for Standardization). 2006. ISO Guide 35:2006. Reference Materials-General and Statistical Principles for Certification. Geneva: International Organization for Standardization.

Khan, I.A., A.R. Afrooz, J.R. Flora, P.A. Schierz, P.L. Ferguson, T. Sabo-Attwood, and N.B. Saleh. 2013. Chirality affects aggregation kinetics of single-walled carbon nanotubes. Environ. Sci. Technol. 47(4):1844-1852.

Kim, H.J., T. Phenrat, R.D. Tilton, and G.V. Lowry. 2012. Effect of kaolinite, silica fines and pH on transport of polymer-modified zero valent iron nano-particles in heterogeneous porous media. J. Colloid Interf. Sci. 370(1):1-10.

Klaine, S.J., P.J. Alvarez, G.E. Batley, T.F. Fernandes, R.D. Handy, D.Y. Lyon, S. Mahendra, M.J. McLaughlin, and J.R. Lead. 2008. Nanomaterials in the environment: Behavior, fate, bioavailability, and effects. Environ. Toxicol. Chem. 27(9):1825-1851.

Kuhlbusch, T.A., C. Asbach, H. Fissan, D. Göhler, and M. Stintz. 2011. Nanoparticle exposure at nanotechnology workplaces: A review. Part Fibre Toxicol. 8(1):22.

Lawrence, J.R., J.J. Dynes, D.R. Korber, G.D. Swerhone, G.G. Leppard, and A.P. Hitchcock. 2012. Monitoring the fate of copper nanoparticles in river biofilms using scanning transmission X-ray microscopy (STXM). Chem. Geol. 39 (329):18-25.

Leitch, M.E., E. Casman, and G.V. Lowry. 2012. Nanotechnology patenting trends through an environmental lens: Analysis of materials and applications. J. Nanopart. Res. 14(11):Art.1283.

Levard, C., E.M. Hotze, G.V. Lowry, and G.E. Brown. 2012. Environmental transformation of silver nanoparticles: Impact on stability and toxicity. Environ. Sci. Technol. 46(13):6900-6914.

Lin, S., Y. Zhao, Z. Ji, J. Ear, C.H. Chang, H. Zhang, C. Low-Kam, K. Yamada, H. Meng, X. Wang, R. Liu, S. Pokhrel, L. Mädler, R. Damoiseaux, T. Xia, H.A. Godwin, S. Lin, and A.E. Nel. 2013. Metal oxides: Zebrafish high-throughput screening to study the impact of dissolvable metal oxide nanoparticles on the hatching enzyme, ZHE1. Small 9(9-10):1775.

Liu, J., J. Katahara, G. Li, S. Coe-Sullivan, and R.H. Hurt. 2012. Degradation products from consumer nanoproducts: A case study on quantum dot lighting. Environ. Sci. Technol. 46(6):3220-3227.

Lombi, E., E. Donner, E. Tavakkoli, T.W. Turney, R. Naidu, B.W. Miller, and K.G. Scheckel. 2012. Fate of zinc oxide nanoparticles during anaerobic digestion of wastewater and post-treatment processing of sewage sludge. Environ. Sci. Technol. 46(16):9089-9096.

Lovern, S.B., and R. Klaper. 2006. *Daphnia magna* mortality when exposed to titanium dioxide and fullerene (C60) nanoparticles. Environ. Toxicol. Chem. 25(4):1132-1137.

Lowry, G.V., K.B. Gregory, S.C. Apte, and J.R. Lead. 2012a. Transformations of nanomaterials in the environment. Environ. Sci. Technol. 46(13):6893-6899.

Lowry, G.V., B.P. Espinasse, A.R. Badireddy, C.J. Richardson, B.C. Reinsch, L.D. Bryant, A.J. Bone, A. Deonarine, S. Chae, M. Therezien, B.P. Colman, H. Hsu-Kim, E.S. Bernhardt, C.W. Matson, and M.R. Wiesner. 2012b. Long-term transformation and fate of manufactured Ag nanoparticles in a simulated large scale freshwater emergent wetland. Environ. Sci. Technol. 46(13):7027-7036.

Lu, S., R. Duffin, C. Poland, P. Daly, F. Murphy, E. Drost, W. Macnee, V. Stone, and K. Donaldson. 2009. Efficacy of simple short-term in vitro assays for predicting the potential of metal oxide nanoparticles to cause pulmonary inflammation. Environ. Health Perspect. 117(2):241-247.

Ma, R., C. Levard, S.M. Marinakos, Y. Cheng, J. Liu, F.M. Michel, G.E. Brown, and G.V. Lowry. 2012. Size-controlled dissolution of organic-coated silver nanoparticles. Environ. Sci. Technol. 46(2):752-759.

Maiorano, G., S. Sabella, B. Sorce, V. Brunetti, M.A. Malvindi, R. Cingolani, and P.P. Pompa. 2010. Effects of cell culture media on the dynamic formation of protein-nanoparticle complexes and influence on the cellular response. ACS Nano 4(12): 7481-7491.

Mandrell, D., L. Truong, C. Jephson, M.R. Sarker, A. Moore, C. Lang, M.T. Simonich, and R.L. Tanguay. 2012. Automated zebrafish chorion removal and single embryo placement: Optimizing throughput of zebrafish developmental toxicity screens. J. Lab Autom. 17(1):66-74.

McNeil, S. 2012. Institutional Needs to Support the Research Enterprise: Coordination, Partnership, and Strategic Planning. Presentation at the Sixth Meeting on a Research Strategy for Environmental, Health, and Safety Aspects of Engineered Nanomaterials, November 7, 2012, Washington, DC.

Meng, H., T. Xia, S. George, and A.E. Nel. 2009. A predictive toxicological paradigm for the safety assessment of nanomaterials. ACS Nano 3(7):1620-1627.

Methner, M., L. Hodson, A. Dames, and C. Geraci. 2010. Nanoparticle Emission Assessment Technique (NEAT) for the identification and measurement of potential inhalation exposure to engineered nanomaterials – Part B: Results from 12 field studies. J. Occup. Environ. Hyg. 7(3):163-176.

Mitrano, D.M., A. Barber, A. Bednar, P. Westerhoff, C.P. Higgins, and J.F. Ranville. 2012. Silver nanoparticle characterization using single particle ICP-MS (SP-ICP-MS) and asymmetrical flow field flow fractionation ICP-MS (AF4-ICP-MS). J. Anal. At. Spectrom. 27(7):1131-1142.

Moghadam, B.Y., W.C. Hou, C. Corredor, P. Westerhoff, and J.D. Posner. 2012. Role of nanoparticle surface functionality in the disruption of model cell membranes. Langmuir 28(47):16318-16326.

Mu, Q., N.S. Hondow, L. Krzeminski, A.P. Brown, L.J. Jeuken, and M.N. Routledge. 2012. Mechanism of cellular uptake of genotoxic silica nanoparticles. Part. Fibre Toxicol. 9:29.

Müller, R., and S. Heinemann. 1989. Surface modeling of microparticles as parenteral systems with high tissue affinity. Pp. 202-214 in Bioadhesion - Possibilities and Future Trends, R. Gurny, and H.E. Junginger, eds. Stuttgart: Wissenschaftliche Verlagsgesellschaft.

Nano Composix. 2012. Material for Nanotoxicology [online]. Available: http://nanocomposix.com/products/nanotoxicology [accessed Jan. 24, 2013].

Nanomaterialregistry. org. 2013. Nanomaterial Registry [online]. Available: https://www.nanomaterialregistry.org/ [accessed Mar. 11, 2013].

Nel, A., T. Xia, H. Meng, X. Wang, S. Lin, Z. Ji, and H. Zhang. 2013. Nanomaterial toxicity testing in the 21st century: Use of a predictive toxicological approach and high-throughput screening. Acc. Chem. Res. 46(3):607-621.

Nguyen, T., B.T. Pellegrin, C. Bernard, S.A. Rabb, P.E. Stutzman, J.M. Gorham, X. Gu, L.L. Yu, and J.W. Chin. 2012. Characterization of surface accumulation and release of nanosilica during irradiation of polymer nanocomposites with ultraviolet light. J. Nanosci. Nanotechnol. 12(8):6202-6215.

NIEHS (National Institute of Environmental Health Science). 2012. NIEHS Centers for Nanotechnology Health Implications Research (NCNHIR) Consortium [online]. Available: (http://www.niehs.nih.gov/research/supported/dert/cospb/programs/nanotech/index.cfm [accessed Apr. 1, 2013].

NIOSH (National Institute for Occupational Safety and Health). 2012a. Project 51: Field Research Team. Pp. 239-243 in Filling the Knowledge Gaps for Safe Nanotechnology in the Workplace: A Progress Report from the NIOSH Nanotechnology Research

Center, 2004-2011. DHHS(NIOSH) 2013-101. U.S. Department of Health and Human Services, Centers for Disease Control and Prevention, National Institute for Occupational Safety and Health. November 2012 [online]. Available: http://www.cdc.gov/niosh/docs/ 2013-101/pdfs/2013-101.pdf [accessed Apr. 1, 2013].

NIOSH (National Institute for Occupational Safety and Health). 2012b. Prevention through Design: Safe Nano Design Workshop, August 14-16, 2012, Albany, NY [online]. Available: http://www.cdc.gov/niosh/topics/ptd/nanoworkshop/default.html [accessed Feb. 2, 2013].

NIST (National Institute of Standards and Technology). 2013a. Material Measurement Laboratory. Standard Reference Materials. SRM Order Request System [online]. Available: https://www-s.nist.gov/srmors/viewTable.cfm?tableid=231 [accessed Jan. 24, 2013].

NIST (National Institute of Standards and Technology). 2013b. Nanotech/Environment, Health, & Safety Portal [online]. Available: http://www.nist.gov/nanotech-environment-health-and-safety-portal.cfm [accessed Apr. 1, 2013].

NNI (U.S. National Nanotechnology Initiative). 2012. Nanotechnology Signature Initiatives. Nano.gov [online]. Available: http://www.nano.gov/signatureinitiatives [accessed Dec. 27, 2012].

NOSH (Nanoparticle Occupational Safety and Health) Consortium. 2007. Nanoparticle Occupational Safety and Health Consortium, Executive Summary [online]. Available: http://www.hse.gov.uk/nanotechnology/consortiumsummary.pdf [accessed Mar. 26, 2013].

Nowack, B., J.F. Ranville, S. Diamond, J.A. Gallego-Urrea, C. Metcalfe, J. Rose, N. Horne, A.A. Koelmans, and S.J. Klaine. 2012. Potential scenarios for nanomaterial release and subsequent alteration in the environment. Environ. Toxicol. Chem. 31(1):50-59.

NRC (National Research Council). 2009. Review of the Federal Strategy for Nanotechnology-Related Environmental, Health, and Safety Research. Washington, DC: National Academies Press.

NRC (National Research Council). 2012. A Research Strategy for the Environmental, Health, and Safety Aspects of Engineered Nanomaterials. Washington, DC: National Academies Press.

NSET (Nanoscale Science, Engineering, and Technology Subcommittee). 2011. Environmental Health and Safety Research Strategy. Subcommittee on Nanoscale Science, Engineering, and Technology, National Science and Technology Council. October 2011 [online]. Available: http://www.nano.gov/sites/default/files/pub_resource/nni_2011_ehs_research_strategy.pdf [accessed Apr. 3, 2013].

NSET (Nanoscale Science, Engineering, and Technology Subcommittee). 2012a. The National Nanotechnology Initiative: Research and Development Leading to a Revolution in Technology and Industry: Supplement to the President's FY 2013 Budget. Subcommittee on Nanoscale Science, Engineering, and Technology, National Science and Technology Council. February 2012 [online]. Available: http://www.nano.gov/sites/default/files/pub_resource/nni_2013_budget_supplement.pdf [accessed Nov. 27, 2012].

NSET (Nanoscale Science, Engineering, and Technology). 2012b. Nanotechnology Signature Initiative. Nanotechnology Knowledge Infrastructure: Enabling National Leadership in Sustainable Design. May 14, 2012 [online]. Available: http://nano.gov/sites/default/files/pub_resource/nki_nsi_white_paper_-_final_for_web.pdf [accessed Jan. 22, 2013].

NSF (National Science Foundation). 2010. Data Management & Sharing Frequently Asked Questions (FAQS). National Science Foundation [online]. Available: http://www.nsf.gov/bfa/dias/policy/dmpfaqs.jsp#1 [accessed Jan. 22, 2013].

Nurkiewicz, T.R., D.W. Porter, A.F. Hubbs, J.L. Cumpston, B.T. Chen, D.G. Frazer, and V. Castranova. 2008. Nanoparticle inhalation augments particle-dependent systemic microvascular dysfunction. Part Fibre Toxicol. 5:1. doi: 10.1186/1743-8977-5-1.

OECD (Organisation for Economic Co-operation and Development). 2008. List of Manufactured Nanomaterials and List of Endpoints for Phase One of the OECD Testing Programme. ENV/JM/MONO(2008)13/REV. Series on the Safety of Manufactured Nanomaterials No. 6 [online]. Available: http://search.oecd.org/officialdocuments/displaydocumentpdf/?cote=env/jm/mono(2008)13/rev&doclanguage=en [accessed July 2, 2013].

OSTP (Office of Science Technology and Policy). 2012. Obama Administration Unveils "Big Data" Initiative: Announces $200 Million in New R&D Investments. Office of Science Technology and Policy, Press Release: May 29, 2012 [online]. Available: http://www.whitehouse.gov/sites/default/files/microsites/ostp/big_data_press_release_final_2.pdf [accessed Jan. 22, 2013].

Ottofuelling, S., F. von der Kammer, and T. Hofmann. 2011. Commercial titanium dioxide nanoparticles in both natural and synthetic water: Comprehensive multidimensional testing and prediction of aggregation behavior. Environ. Sci. Technol. 45(23):10045-10052.

PCAST (President's Council of Advisors on Science and Technology). 2010. Report to the President and Congress on the Third Assessment of the National Nanotechnology Initiative. March 2010 [online]. Available: http://www.whitehouse.gov/sites/default/files/microsites/ostp/pcast-nano-report.pdf [accessed Dec. 20, 2012].

PCAST (President's Council of Advisors on Science and Technology). 2012. Report to the President and Congress on the Fourth Assessment of the National Nanotechnology Initiative. April 2012 [online]. Available: http://nano.gov/sites/default/files/pub_resource/pcast_2012_nanotechnology_final.pdf [accessed Mar.11, 2013].

PEN (Project on Emerging Nanotechnologies). 2013. Consumer Products. An Inventory of Nanotechnology-based Consumer Products Currently on the Market [online]. Available: http://www.nanotechproject.org/inventories/consumer/ [accessed July 2, 2013].

Perez, R.A., B.E. Albero, E. Miguel, J.L. Tadeo, and C. Sanchez-Brunete. 2013. A rapid procedure for the determination of C60 and C70 fullerenes in soil and sediments by ultrasound-assisted extraction and HPLC-UV. Anal. Sci. 29(5):533-538.

Pettit, M.E., and J.R. Lead. 2013. Minimum physicochemical characterization requirements for nanomaterial regulation. Environ. Int. 52:41-50.

Phenrat, T., H.J. Kim, F. Fagerlund, T. Illangasekare, and G.V. Lowry. 2010. Empirical correlations to estimate agglomeration, deposition, and transport of polyelectrolyte-modified Fe(0) nanoparticles at high particle concentration in saturated porous media. J. Contam. Hydrol. 118(3-4):152-164.

Priester, J.H.,Y. Ge, R.E. Mielke, A.M. Horst, S.C. Moritz, K. Espinosa, J. Gelb, S.L. Walker, R.M. Nisbet, Y.J. An, J.P. Schimel, R.G. Palmer, J.A. Hernandez-Viezcas, L. Zhao, J.L. Gardea-Torresdey, and P.A. Holden. 2012. Soybean susceptibility to manufactured nanomaterials with evidence for quality and soil fertility interruption. Proc. Natl. Acad. Sci. USA 109(37):E2451–E2456.

Rhoads, K.P., D.J. Phares, A.S. Wexler, and M.V. Johnston. 2003. Size-resolved ultrafine particle composition analysis, 1. Atlanta. J. Geophy. Res. 108(D7):8418.

Richman, E.K., and J.E. Hutchison. 2009. The nanomaterial characterization bottleneck. ACS Nano 3(9): 2441-2446.

Robichaud, C.O., A.E. Uyar, M.R. Darby, L.G. Zucker, and M.R. Wiesner. 2009. Estimates of upper bounds and trends in nano-TiO2 production as a basis for exposure assessment. Environ. Sci. Technol. 43(12):4227-4233.

Roebben, G., S. Ramirez-Garcia, V.A. Hackley, M. Roesslein, F. Klaessig, V. Kestens, I. Lynch, C.M. Garner, A. Rawle, A. Elder, V. L. Colvin, W. Kreyling, H.F. Krug, Z.A. Lewicka, S. McNeil, A. Nel, A. Patri, P. Wick, M. Wiesner, T. Xia, G. Oberdörster, and K.A. Dawson. 2011. Interlaboratory comparison of size and surface charge measurements on nanoparticles prior to biological impact assessment. J. Nanopart. Res. 13(7):2675-2687.

Rushton, E.K., J. Jiang, S.S. Leonard, S. Eberly, V. Castranova, P. Biswas, A. Elder, X. Han, R. Gelein, J. Finkelstein, and G. Oberdörster. 2010. Concept of assessing nanoparticle hazards considering nanoparticle dosimetric and chemical/biological response metrics. J. Toxicol. Environ. Health A 73(5):445-461.

Sayes, C.M., K.L. Reed, and D.B. Warheit. 2007. Assessing toxicity of fine and nanoparticles: Comparing in vitro measurements to in vivo pulmonary toxicity profiles. Toxicol. Sci. 97(1):163-180.

Sayes, C.M., K.L. Reed, S. Subramoney, L. Abrams, and D.B. Warheit. 2009. Can in vitro assays substitute for in vivo studies in assessing the pulmonary hazards of fine and nanoscale materials? J. Nanopart. Res. 11(2):421-431.

Schierz, A., A.N. Parks, K.M. Washburn, T.G. Chandler, and P.L. Ferguson. 2012. Characterization and quantitative analysis of single-walled carbon nanotubes in the aquatic environment using near-infrared fluorescence spectroscopy. Environ. Sci. Technol. 46(22):12262-12271.

Slikker, W., Jr., M.E. Andersen, M.S. Bogdanffy, J.S. Bus, S.D. Cohen, R.B. Conolly, R.M. David, N.G. Doerrer, D.C. Dorman, D.W. Gaylor, D. Hattis, J.M. Rogers, R.W. Setzer, J.A. Swenberg, and K. Wallace. 2004. Dose-dependent transitions in mechanisms of toxicity: Case studies. Toxicol. Appl. Pharmacol. 201(3):226-294.

Stone, V., B. Nowack, A. Baun, N. van den Brink, F. von der Kammer, M. Dusinska, R. Handy, S. Hankin, M. Hassellöv, E. Joner, and T.F. Fernandes. 2010. Nanomaterials for environmental studies: Classification reference material issues, and strategies for physio-chemical characterization. Sci. Total Environ. 408(7):1745-1754.

Thomas, C.R., S. George, A.M. Horst, Z. Ji, R.J. Miller, J.R. Peralta-Videa, T. Xia, S. Pokhrel, L. Mädler, J.L. Gardea-Torresdey, P.A. Holden, A.A. Keller, H.S. Lenihan, A.E. Nel, and J.I. Zink. 2011. Nanomaterials in the environment: From materials to high-throughput screening to organisms. ACS Nano. 5(1):13-20.

Thomas, D.G., S. Gaheen, S.L. Harper, M. Fritts, F. Klaessig, E. Hahn-Dantona, D. Paik, S. Pan, G.A. Stafford, E.T. Freund, J.D. Klemm, and N.A. Baker. 2013. ISA-TAB-Nano: A specification for sharing nanomaterial research data in spreadsheet-based format. BMC Biotechnol. 13:2, doi:10.1186/1472-6750-13-2.

Thomas, R.S., M.B. Black, L. Li, E. Healy, T.M. Chu, W. Bao, M.E. Andersen, and R.D. Wolfinger. 2012a. A comprehensive statistical analysis of predicting in vivo hazard using high-throughput in vitro screening. Toxicol. Sci. 128(2):398-417.

Thomas, R.S., M.B. Black, L. Li, E. Healy, T.M. Chu, W. Bao, M.E. Andersen, and R.D. Wolfinger. 2012b. Response to "incorporating biological, chemical, and toxicological knowledge into predictive models of toxicity". Toxicol. Sci. 130(2):442-443.

Tsai, S.J., A. Ashter, E. Ada, J.L. Mead, C.F. Barry, and M.J. Ellenbecker. 2008. Airborne nanoparticle release associated with the compounding of nanocomposite using nanoalumina as fillers. J. Aerosol Air Qual. Res. 8(2):160-177.

Tsai, S.J., M. Hofmann, M. Hallock, E. Ada, J. Kong, and M. Ellenbecker. 2009. Characterization and evaluation of nanoparticle release during the synthesis of single-walled and multiwalled carbon nanotubes by chemical vapor deposition. Environ. Sci. Technol. 43(15):6017-6023.

Tsai, S.J., D. White, H. Rodriguez, C.E. Munoz, C.Y. Huang, C.J. Tsai, C. Barry, and M.J. Ellenbecker. 2012. Exposure assessment and engineering control strategies for airborne nanoparticles: An application to emissions from nanocomposite compounding processes. J. Nanopart. Res. 14(7):Art. 989.

Unrine, J.M., W.A. Shoults-Wilson, O. Zhurbich, P.M. Bertsch, and O.V. Tsyusko. 2012. Trophic transfer of Au nanoparticles from soil along a simulated terrestrial food chain. Environ. Sci. Technol. 46(17):9753-9760.

Verma, A., and F. Stellacci. 2009. Effect of surface properties on nanoparticle–cell interactions. Small 6(1):12-21.

von der Kammer, F., P.L. Ferguson, P.A. Holden, A. Masion, K.R. Rogers, S.J. Klaine, A.A. Koelmans, N. Horne, and J.M. Unrine. 2012. Analysis of engineered nanomaterials in complex matrices (environment & biota): General considerations and conceptual case studies. Environ. Toxicol. Chem. 31(1):32-49.

Walczyk, D., F.B. Bombelli, M.P. Monopoli, I. Lynch, and K.A. Dawson. 2010. What the cell "sees" in bionanoscience. J. Am Chem. Soc. 132(16):5761-5768.

Wang, H., R.L. Wick, and B. Xing. 2009. Toxicity of nanoparticulate and bulk ZnO, Al_2O_3 and TiO_2 to the nematode *Caenorhabditis elegans*. Environ. Pollut. 157(4):1171-1177.

Wang, J., C. Asbach, H. Fissan, T. Hülser, T. Kuhlbusch, D. Thompson, and D. Pui. 2011. How can nanobiotechnology oversight advance science and industry: Examples from environmental, health, and safety studies of nanoparticles (nano-EHS). J. Nanopart. Res. 13(4):1373-1387.

Wang, S., J. Kurepa., and J.A. Smalle. 2011. Ultra-small TiO_2 nanoparticles disrupt microtubular networks in *Arabidopsis thaliana*. Plant Cell Environ. 34(5):811-820.

Wang, Y., P.K. Hopke, L. Sun, D.C. Chalupa, and M.J. Utell. 2011. Laboratory and field testing of an automated atmospheric particle-bound reactive oxygen species sampling-analysis system. J. Toxicol. 2011:Art.419476, doi:10.1155/2011/419476.

Warheit, D.B., C.M. Sayes, and K.L. Reed. 2009. Nanoscale and fine zinc oxide particles: Can in vitro assays accurately forecast lung hazards following inhalation exposures? Environ. Sci. Technol. 43(20):7939-7945.

Werlin, R., J.H. Priester, R.E. Mielke, S. Krämer, S. Jackson, P.K. Stoimenov, G.D. Stucky, G.N. Cherr, E. Orias, and P.A. Holden. 2011. Biomagnification of cadmium selenide quantum dots in a simple experimental microbial food chain. Nat. Nanotechnol. 6(1):65-71.

Westerhoff, P., and B. Nowack. 2013. Searching for global descriptors of engineered nanomaterial fate and transport in the environment. Acc. Chem. Res. 46(3):844-853.

Westerhoff, P., G. Song, K. Hristovski, and M.A. Kiser. 2011. Occurrence and removal of titanium at full scale wastewater treatment plants: Implications for TiO_2 nanomaterials. J. Environ. Monit. 13(5):1195-1203.

Wiesner, M.R., G.V. Lowry, K.L. Jones, M.F. Hochella, Jr., R.T. Di Giulio, E. Casman, and E.S. Bernhardt. 2009. Decreasing uncertainties in assessing environmental exposure, risk, and ecological implications of nanomaterials. Environ. Sci. Technol. 43(17):6458- 6462.

Wohlleben, W., S. Brill, M.W. Meier, M. Mertler, G. Cox, S. Hirth, B. von Vacano, V. Strauss, S. Treumann, K. Wiench, L. Ma-Hock, and R. Landsiedel. 2011. On the lifecycle of nanocomposites: Comparing released fragments and their in-vivo hazards from three release mechanisms and four nanocomposites. Small 7(16):2384-2395.

Xiao, Y., and M.R. Wiesner. 2012. Characterization of surface hydrophobicity of engineered nanoparticles. J. Hazard. Mater. 215-216:146-151.

Yang, Y., J.M. Mathieu, S. Chattopadhyay, J.T. Miller, T. Wu, T. Shibata, W. Guo, and P.J. Alvarez. 2012. Defense mechanisms of *Pseudomonas aeruginosa* PAO1 against quantum dots and their released heavy metals. ACS Nano 6(7):6091-6098.

Zhang, H., Z. Ji, T, Xia, H. Meng, C. Low-Kam, R. Liu, S. Pokhrel, S. Lin, X. Wang, Y.P. Liao, M. Wang, L. Li, R. Rallo, R. Damoiseaux, D. Telesca, L. Mädler, Y. Cohen, J.I. Zink, and A.E. Nel. 2012. Use of metal oxide nanoparticle band gap to develop a predictive paradigm for oxidative stress and acute pulmonary inflammation. ACS Nano. 6(5):4349-4368.

Zhu, M.T., G.J. Nie, H. Meng, T. Xia, A. Nel, and Y.L. Zhao. 2013. Physicochemical properties determine nanomaterial cellular uptake, transport, and fate. Acc. Chem. Res. 46(3):622-631.

4

Getting to Green

INTRODUCTION

The research enterprise that is investigating potential risks to human health and ecosystems posed by engineered nanomaterials (ENMs) engages a broad and multidisciplinary array of stakeholders, including researchers, the industrial sector, and the public at large. The success of research in this domain, as in others, depends on identifying—through stakeholder engagement—the most critical questions that need to be addressed; networking in the United States and internationally among investigators in government, academe, and industry; developing standards for analyses and reference materials; using uniform terminology and data descriptions; capturing data in an accessible, quality-assured database; and continuing to refine research methods. Figure 4-1 represents the committee's construct for a successful research enterprise in the potential environmental, health, and safety (EHS) risks posed by ENMs. The figure describes the interrelated and interdependent research activities that are driven by the evolving production of ENMs. A critical output is an evaluation of risk that informs decision-making on ENMs. The diagram is aspirational, offering a vision for an integrated and strategic system for developing data that will provide for the characterization of ENMs, refinement of experimental methods, and support for model development to predict and then prevent and manage risks associated with new ENMs. Many of the elements are already in place, but such an overall framework has not yet been articulated. The committee considers that the development and integration of the elements of such a framework are essential for advancing the progress necessary to "get to green" on the committee's identified research priorities. Similar frameworks have been articulated for other research endeavors; for example, a recent report on "precision medicine" by the National Research Council provided a theoretical framework for translating advances in biomedical research into clinical practice (NRC 2011; Figure 3-1).

84   *Research Progress on EHS Aspects of Engineered Nanomaterials*

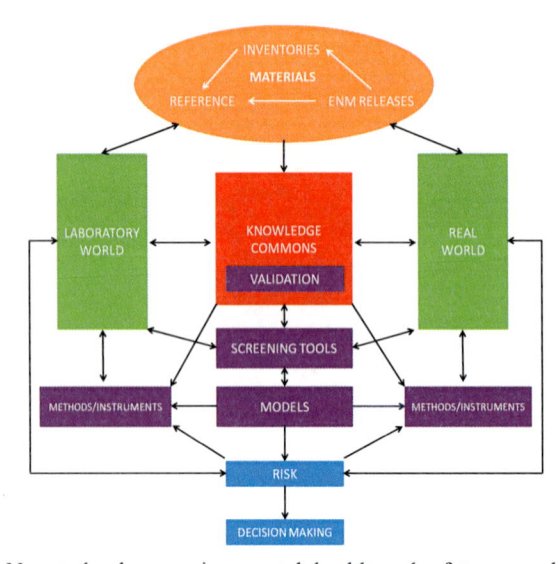

FIGURE 4-1 Nanotechnology environmental, health, and safety research enterprise. The diagram shows the integrated and interdependent research activities that are driven by the production of ENMs. The production of ENMs is captured by the orange oval, labeled "materials", which includes reference materials, ENM releases, and inventories. (An inventory is a quantitative estimate of the location and amounts of nanomaterials produced or current production capacity, including the properties of the nanomaterial.) The knowledge commons (red box) is the locus for collaborative development of methods, models, and materials, and for archiving and sharing data. The "laboratory world" and "real world" (green boxes) feed into the knowledge commons. The laboratory world comprises process-based and mechanism-based research that is directed at understanding the physical, chemical, and biologic properties or processes that are most critical for assessing exposures and hazards and hence risk (NRC 2012, p. 55). The "real world" includes complex systems research involving observational studies that examine the effects of ENMs on people and ecosystems. The purple boxes capture the range of methods, tools, models, and instruments that support generation of research in the laboratory world, the real world, and the knowledge commons.

Of necessity, Figure 4-1 provides a simplified vision of a complex system of knowledge creation and use, but each of its elements is critical. The system places research into two broad domains: "laboratory world", process-based or mechanism-based research directed at the "critical elements of nanomaterial interactions" (a central component of the committee's conceptual framework; see Chapter 1); and "real world", systems research involving observational studies that examine the effects of ENMs on complex experimental models of human health and ecosystems. The research is supported by the availability of materials (reference materials, materials from inventories developed with industry input, and materials released and modified through their value chain and life

Getting to Green 85

cycle), analytic methods and instrumentation, and a "knowledge commons", which is central to this schema. The knowledge commons incorporates a standard nomenclature, data classifications, and storage of data with sufficient detail to facilitate informed modeling. The success of the research enterprise requires that all researchers place their data (in a compatible form) in a data-management commons that is supported by appropriate hardware and software.

"Models" of many types are inherent in Figure 4-1. For example, some models will be used to estimate exposures of human populations and ecosystems to ENMs across their value chains and life cycles. Predictive models need to be developed to anticipate risks posed by ENMs. Such models require validation, which will be facilitated by an iterative process that involves data access through the knowledge commons. "Screening tools" will be needed to generate data that can be used to establish priorities for knowledge creation that in turn can be used to formulate models to predict risks posed by new ENMs. Such knowledge generation will be developed in an iterative fashion that draws on research results from mechanistic and complex systems of research.

Figure 4-1 shows the relationship between the research activities and risk, which in turn inform a broad range of decision-making by diverse stakeholders, including regulators, manufacturers, and the public. Models provide the bridge from research findings to risk estimation and characterization of uncertainty. The estimation of risk is iterative. The overall research process provides feedback to materials generation with the goal of reducing the potential risk presented by ENMs and the products that they enable.

Several features of Figure 4-1 merit emphasis. The relationships among its components are dynamic, and there are multiple feedbacks (represented by the arrows) among them. The success of the research enterprise hinges on the creation of a knowledge commons and engagement of the broad community of researchers who are addressing potential risks to human health and ecosystems. It also requires stakeholder engagement, particularly of the manufacturing sector, to ensure that the materials studied reflect those in use and that the most critical research questions are addressed. Leadership in its development and stewardship of its maintenance are also essential.

In the discussion below, the committee analyzes the findings of Chapter 3 in the context of the flow of activities in the nanotechnology EHS research enterprise (Figure 4-1), examining pathways to advance research and mechanisms to improve implementation of the enterprise with an eye to "getting to green" on the committee's indicators (Boxes 3-1 and 3-2). First, research progress is considered, and the steps needed to advance the research are described. The discussion is divided into six major subjects as reflected in the research enterprise: nanomaterial processes and mechanisms, material sources and development of reference materials, model development, methods and instrumentation, the knowledge commons, and nanomaterial interactions in complex systems. Then, progress on mechanisms to ensure implementation of the research is evaluated, and the steps needed to advance implementation of the research are discussed.

FUNDAMENTAL PROCESSES THAT AFFECT NANOMATERIAL EXPOSURE AND HAZARD

The committee's first report identified the need for research on cross-cutting processes that affect both exposure and hazard (see Figure 1-1). The research entails identifying fundamental processes, typically through laboratory experiments. A description of the processes is needed to develop general and predictive capabilities to assess risks that move beyond case-by-case evaluations of ENMs. The process-based activities described in Figure 4-1 are enabled by continual development of methods and instrumentation. The experimental approach is updated through understanding of material properties and the evolving physical, chemical, and biologic processes that affect exposure and hazard. Hypothesized properties or mechanisms can be scrutinized in well-defined laboratory experiments and in observations of ENM behavior in complex systems, from in vivo experiments to models of ecosystem interactions in microcosms, mesocosms, and field observations. Boundaries between well-defined laboratory and complex systems may be blurred, but the key contrast is that between a reductionist approach to unraveling elements that may affect organisms, populations, and ecosystems and holistic examination of ENMs in complex systems. Both approaches are needed, and they are complementary.

Ideally, the agenda for process-based research is influenced in part by findings on the extent to which research reduces uncertainty in the understanding of potential risks. Reducing uncertainty requires updating of models to increase our understanding of risks to human health and ecosystems, motivated in part by needs of stakeholders (whether workers producing ENMs or consumers of ENM-enabled products). Information generated from process-based research influences how ENMs are produced, including considerations of life-cycle risks and relevant reference materials for conducting studies.

Substantial progress (green) has been made in exploring mechanisms that control the dynamics and transformation of ENMs. However, only moderate (yellow) progress has been achieved in development of methods to quantify effects of ENMs in experimental systems; this level of progress may reflect the complex nature of in vivo experiments and the need for model development and verification. The roles of methods and instrumentation in understanding mechanisms of ENM transformations, distribution, and effects highlight the state of progress in developing methods for ENM characterization and detection in relevant media; and this indicator has been noted as green. That stands in strong contrast with the relatively limited progress made in translating methods to readily available instrumentation for characterizing ENM properties and their transformations; this indicator was denoted as red, and the lack of progress represents a key impediment to advancing understanding of processes and mechanisms.

Steps to Ensure Progress Toward Elucidating Mechanisms

Continued, vigorous activity to elucidate mechanisms of ENM interactions with organisms and ecosystems is critical for reaching the long-term goal of predicting ENM effects. The ability to make such predictions will allow evaluation of risks posed by ENMs at the design stage, in model predictions, and in validated screening assays. The interdependences described in Figure 4-1 and the state of research progress indicated in Box 3-1 imply that continued progress in understanding mechanisms of ENM behavior will require advances in instrument development and increased availability of up-to-date instrumentation to researchers. Another key impediment to progress is the relative lack of a data-integration infrastructure and of validated models that reflect field-tested theories.

NANOMATERIAL SOURCES AND DEVELOPMENT OF REFERENCE MATERIALS

The committee's nanotechnology EHS research strategy is driven by the need to assess potential risks associated with the accelerating production of new ENMs and materials that are present in an increasing number of products. As shown in Figure 4-1, ENMs are the central element of nanotechnology-related research studies in the knowledge commons, the laboratory world (mechanism-driven research), and the real world (investigations in complex systems). Three primary types of ENMs (shown in the figure) are the focus of these studies: reference materials, nanomaterial-enabled products (inventories), and released nanoscale species (ENM releases). Reference materials were described in the committee's first report and include individual ENMs and libraries of ENMs that are used to conduct targeted studies to answer EHS-research questions. Nanomaterial-enabled products are ENMs found in the inventory of substances being incorporated into commercial products. ENM releases are materials that come from products that may be transformed as they are released.

The need for appropriately designed and adequately characterized ENMs was highlighted in the first report (NRC 2012, pp. 181-182). That report called for

Developing nanomaterials and libraries:

- Extent of development of libraries of well-characterized nanomaterials, including those prevalent in commerce and reference and standard materials.

Providing feedback to inform the design of appropriate nanomaterials:

- Development of inventories of current and near-term production of nanomaterials.
- Development of inventories of intended use of nanomaterials and value-chain transfers.
- Identification of critical release points along the value chain.
- Identification of benchmark (positive and negative) and reference materials, for use in such studies and measurement tools and methods to estimate exposure and dose in those complex systems.

- In addition to those direct calls for action, the need for nanomaterials to support other research priorities was implicit as described elsewhere in this chapter. Appropriate ENMs are needed to carry out research that will generate data needed to populate the knowledge commons, to develop new methods and instruments, to conduct mechanistic studies, and to perform investigations in complex media.
- Research to characterize ENM production and releases along the value chain was generally considered to show moderate progress (yellow). However, very little progress was considered to have occurred in modeling releases along the value chain (denoted as red). Moreover, the lack of a systematic *process* for collecting information on the production of ENMs and the lack of a process for providing feedback from the research enterprise to improve the sustainability of ENMs together limit the pace of the entire research enterprise.
- As discussed in Chapter 3, progress in developing ENMs for study was evaluated as some to little (rated either yellow or red). In particular, little to no progress was considered to have occurred in developing benchmark (for positive and negative controls) and reference materials for metrology. The nanotechnology EHS-research enterprise has mostly relied on commonly available nanoparticles to conduct most studies. These particles, typically produced to evaluate their use in specific applications or produced as commercially available research samples, are largely categorized by core material. The vast majority of the studies have been conducted on a relatively small number of core species, including carbon nanomaterials (tubes, fullerenes, and graphene), metals (primarily silver and gold), metal oxides (primarily zinc oxide, titanium dioxide, cerium oxide), and polymeric materials. There is no process to determine which nanomaterials should have high priority for development on the basis of the needs for mechanistic studies or investigations of materials in complex systems. To move high-priority research toward green, additional effort and coordination are required to develop appropriate nanomaterial libraries. Similarly, the lack of a systematic *process* for collecting information needed to create a picture of nanomaterial production along the value chain limits the pace of research required to conduct risk evaluations and the feedback needed to improve nanomaterial properties from EHS and sustainability perspectives.

Steps to Ensure Progress Toward Providing Reference Materials

The lack of availability of ENMs for research and the limits of our knowledge of commercial ENM production quantities and formats create a critical-path challenge in advancing nanotechnology EHS research. Important elements for advancing the development and distribution of reference nanomaterials for research and analytic purposes include

- *A mechanism to identify and set priorities among nanomaterials and libraries for development.* Developing precisely defined and characterized reference materials is expensive and time-consuming. Sustainable approaches are needed to set priorities among materials for development and distribution to researchers.
- *Material descriptors and other nomenclature to distinguish properly between different nanomaterial samples.* Appropriate and standardized material descriptors need to be adopted and used. Without such descriptors, the specificity or precision with which nanomaterials are designed, developed, and shared will not be sufficient, particularly for developing the knowledge commons. This is one aspect of the ontology that needs to be developed for ENMs.
- *Improved synthesis and purification methods.* Once nanomaterials are identified for research purposes, the synthesis and purification methods to produce them may need to be developed. Although some methods have been developed for synthesis of specific classes of nanomaterials, new methods need to be developed for other nanomaterials that have been identified for development.
- *Collaborations among scientists who are studying mechanisms and complex systems so that materials for these studies can be optimized.* The production of a reference material or library is only the beginning of its development. Reference nanomaterials require further optimization through collaboration among material developers and users (for example, to optimize handling protocols or for in situ monitoring of the nanomaterials).
- *Instrumentation for rapid characterization of reference materials.* Although there has been progress in developing instrumentation and protocols for characterization of pristine, synthesized nanoparticles in the laboratory, new methods and approaches are needed to accelerate routine characterization. For example, laboratory-scale, small-angle x-ray scattering can be used to reduce the number of artifacts during analysis and reduce the time for characterization from hours (or days) to minutes relative to transmission electron microscopy.
- *Instrumentation to characterize complex nanoscale species (that is, materials of unknown origin, mixtures, and released materials).* Each of these material classes presents challenges to characterizing their structure, composition, and purity—substantial barriers to studying their effects on health and the environment. Those barriers reflect the lack of information on the starting composition and structure of the materials and the lack of knowledge of their history.

- *Mechanisms and incentives for collecting information.* Information management plans and appropriate research infrastructure are needed to create a process for collecting information on nanomaterial production and uses along the value chain.

Steps to Ensure Progress Toward Characterizing Commercial Sources of Nanomaterials

- *Greater investment in research at the interface between the physical sciences, social sciences, and business.* A full understanding of potential risks along the value chain requires broad and multidisciplinary expertise that will bridge physical and social sciences and engage the commercial sector. The critical topics include trends in nanomaterial production, value-chain analysis, and human behavior in relation to use of products that contain ENMs and the potential for exposures along the value chain and throughout the life cycle. An improved understanding of those factors is needed as a starting point for modeling nanomaterial exposure along the value chain.

MODEL DEVELOPMENT

A key outcome of the integration of data and information contained in the knowledge commons is development of a suite of models. The models allow the application of new methods and instruments that reflect thinking regarding hypothesis testing and assessment. Such models may be used to predict physical characteristics of ENMs, outcomes of toxicity testing, and exposure potential in complex systems. In their initial forms, the models represent working assumptions that are refined with additional data. As confidence in a model increases, validation studies that involve comparisons of model outputs with results from experimental systems that use benchmark or unknown ENMs can be conducted. The process of data integration and model formulation and validation informs risk assessment. Given adequate knowledge, refined and validated models allow prediction of potential hazards associated with exposure to ENMs throughout their life cycle and value chain.

Mechanistic models should provide the greatest long-term benefit to the EHS nanotechnology research community with regard to anticipating risks. However identifying the critical elements of nanomaterial-environment and nanomaterial-biota interactions is a significant undertaking and will take time to develop. There is a near term need to predict behaviors of nanomaterials in relevant environmental and biologic matrices. Empirical predictive models that are parameterized appropriately (for example, partition coefficients between nanomaterials and bacteria in wastewater treatment plants or approximate dissolution rates and half times in specific media) may be sufficient to approximate behaviors of ENMs in selected matrices. The forms of these predictive models, their parameters, and appropriate assays to measure the values for these parameters in selected environmental and biologic media are still needed (Hou et al. 2013; Westerhoff and Nowack 2013).

As described in Chapter 3, several indicators of research progress involve successful model development. They include qualitative and quantitative models to characterize the origins and releases of ENMs into the environment. The ability to address potential releases, transformations, environmental concentrations, and exposures was highlighted previously. Efforts appear to be focused on specific release points and routes of exposures (see examples in Chapter 3); progress in this indicator is considered to be minimal (red in Table 3-1). Progress is hampered by a lack of information on ENMs in the value chain for particular ENM-containing products and a lack of data from experimental studies to inform modeling efforts on fate and transport in the environment. In another research indicator in Chapter 3, progress toward the use of experimental research results in initial modeling efforts for predicting ENM behavior in complex biologic and environmental settings was considered minimal (red). Because ENM behavior will be influenced by the characteristics of the material and the properties of the system into which it is released, development of integrated models will be important. Those efforts have been limited by the lack of resources for conducting long-term fate and transport studies in complex environmental systems, such as mesocosms, or in in vivo studies. An additional limitation is the absence of a knowledge commons in which research data from multiple studies can be integrated with other information and model outputs to be used in these complex, initial models. Some individual efforts were identified, but they lack the consistency in approaches and interoperability of data that is needed to support effective model development. The efforts also suffer from a focus on a small number of ENMs, which hinders the development of more widely applicable predictive models.

Steps to Ensure Progress Toward Validated Models for Nanomaterial Risk

Getting to green in the development of predictive models requires substantial development of data from mechanistic and complex system studies and characterization of physical properties of a variety of ENMs in different complex environments. Initial working models will require iterative development as data emerge. Early outputs of the models can determine future data needs and influence decisions about experimental approaches and instrumentation needs. Data should be collected with consideration of future data integration and modeling efforts. Input of the data into a knowledge commons is needed to allow a wide array of investigators to engage in modeling efforts. Validation studies that use families of materials in various complex environments will be required. Models for assessing hazard, exposure, and risk will depend on the data sources, and appropriate information management and integration will help to produce a more coordinated and focused approach for addressing EHS aspects of ENMs.

METHODS AND INSTRUMENTATION

The need for methods and instrumentation to characterize ENMs in relevant media is pervasive in the nanotechnology EHS research enterprise. Methods and instrumentation are defined here as the tools required to detect and to characterize ENMs and their properties in relevant media. Toxicity testing and other screening assays are discussed later in this chapter. Not surprisingly, the need for characterization and detection methods is apparent in the four primary cross-cutting research categories identified in the committee's first report: adaptive research and knowledge for accelerating research progress and providing rapid feedback, quantifying and characterizing the origins of nanomaterial releases, processes affecting hazard and exposure, and nanomaterial interactions in complex systems. Progress in the development and validation of the methods and instrumentation needed for those categories ranged from green to red. That range reflects the different characterization needs and scenarios identified. For example, methods and instrumentation needed to characterize newly manufactured ENMs and their important properties (with a few notable exceptions discussed below) in a well-characterized and relatively simple medium (such as deionized water or simple physiologic buffer) are well established. The variations in ENM properties (such as size) measured with different techniques are recognized and can be documented with appropriate methods and metadata. Therefore, progress toward development of methods and instrumentation in well-controlled, simple media is designated green.

However, there are fewer reliable methods for characterizing ENMs in increasingly complex and less well-characterized media (such as blood and natural waters) because complex nonequilibrium interactions between the ENMs and the components of the medium can lead to measurement artifacts or even preclude measurement. For example, measuring the size of ENMs in fluid with light-scattering methods and identifying a specific material with electron microscopy are difficult in the presence of other background particles. Some research has been initiated to modify existing techniques (for example, x-ray absorption spectroscopy [Lombi et al. 2012]) or to develop new ones (for example, hyperspectral imaging [Badireddy et al. 2012] and single-particle ICP-MS [Mitrano et al. 2012]) to address the shortcomings. Thus, the committee designated progress in developing methods and instrumentation as yellow in "quantifying and characterizing nanomaterial releases" (NRC 2012, p. 181) and "processes affecting both hazard and exposure" (p. 149). Progress in those research categories depends on the ability to measure ENM properties in complex media and progress in the development of methods and instrumentation to track, detect, and characterize ENMs in complex environments (such as soil or wastewater in which the origins of ENMs and the composition of the solution are unknown and ENMs are present in very low concentrations) has been particularly poor. New instrumentation for single-particle measurements has also seen little progress, so this indicator was denoted red.

In summary, there has been progress in adapting existing tools for use in well-defined systems, but considerably less progress has been achieved as the complexity of the medium has increased or in understanding the properties of individual particles. The lack of adequate methods and instrumentation for tracking, and for detection and characterization of ENMs in complex systems hinders research progress in many critical research fields. The inability to isolate single-particles also constrains our ability to determine mechanistically how ENM properties affect their behavior.

Steps to Improve Progress in Methods and Instrumentation Development

Advancing research requires methods and instrumentation for measuring key properties of ENMs, particularly in complex media. There are several critical needs. First, the average properties of the ENMs in relevant complex biologic and environmental media and in the matrices in which they will be used need to be quantified and characterized. Second, the properties of single particles need to be measured so that specific ENM properties can be associated with observed behavior and effects. Third, there needs to be an ability to track ENMs in complex media and organisms (for example, using isotopic signatures or radio-labeled materials). Fourth, methods to extract ENMs from complex matrices or to perform in-situ measurements are needed. Finally, the methods developed need to be sensitive enough to be operable at the very low concentrations of ENMs expected in the biologic and environmental samples.

There are two principal challenges in quantifying and characterizing the average properties of ENMs in complex biologic and environmental matrices: the low concentrations of the ENMs in the matrices and the unknown history of the ENMs before analysis. That is important because ENMs in samples taken from organisms or the environment may undergo transformations that change their properties and make it difficult to quantify and laborious to characterize them with existing methods. Released materials in their environments cannot be characterized without appropriate measurement and characterization methods. Appropriate methods to isolate nanoparticles from complex matrices (such as field-flow fractionation or liquid extractions) and appropriate detectors for measuring chemical composition, speciation, and other relevant properties (such as charge) need to be developed. Spectroscopic methods, such as x-ray absorption spectroscopy and near infared fluorescence spectroscopy, that eliminate the need to isolate ENMs from complex matrices (such as soil and tissue), also need additional development. Spectroscopic methods require greater spatial resolution and sensitivity to characterize and quantify ENMs at low environmental and in vivo concentrations. The ability to monitor the transformations of ENMs directly in a matrix in real time would improve our understanding of the critical processes that affect ENM behavior. That will probably require instrumentation that has not been and is not being developed.

Single-particle characterization techniques are needed to determine how specific ENM properties affect their behavior. Most ENMs are polydisperse and have varied properties, such as size, crystal defects, and chemical composition. Exposure to ENMs is typically to a distribution of ENMs with known *average* properties. Single-particle characterization methods would allow one to isolate how the specific features of an ENM affect its behavior. Such methods as tethering ENMs to a transmission electronic microscopy grid can enable tracking behavior of individual particles. Better spatial resolution of microscopy and spectroscopy methods will also allow characterization of individual ENMs.

A critical research need that cuts across exposure and effects research is the characterization of the properties of adsorbed macromolecules on ENMs, including the structure of the macromolecule and the outer surface layers of the ENMs. That information is needed to describe properties and changes of ENMs in relevant biologic and environmental media. It is also a prerequisite to development of appropriate models for predicting ENM behavior in complex systems (such as biouptake models) and effects. It is an extremely challenging task, especially in complex media, and will probably require new instrumentation with spatial resolution adequate for focusing on single particles and initial development in well-characterized systems before application in more complex media.

Another important component of this research is the ability to determine critical release points along the value chain and to identify exposed populations. Therefore, characterization in relevant complex matrices requires methods for characterizing ENMs and transformations in the matrix in which the ENMs are used. The matrix may affect the ENM properties that are used to measure pristine ENMs (such as fluorescence or absorption at a specific wavelength); therefore, development of new methods or validation of existing methods is needed to detect and characterize ENMs released from their matrices.

It is important that the measured properties and characteristics of transformed ENMs be captured in the knowledge commons. That requires an ontology for describing such properties as the adsorbed macromolecular layer. Placing such data in the knowledge commons will allow the community to share them and to develop and update models for describing the behavior of the ENMs in complex environments.

INFORMATICS: THE KNOWLEDGE COMMONS

In Figure 4-1, the knowledge commons performs three functions. The first is to broaden participation in the development and validation of predictive models, particularly risk models. To accomplish that, more effective communication is needed among those engaged in reductionist science (the laboratory world) at the left of the figure, those engaged in integrative science (the real world) at the right, and the information on materials at the top of the figure. Model development via the knowledge commons would be hosted in a collaborative environment with access to both processed and raw experimental data and data from other, lower-level computations and simulations. The iterative model validation process would lead to publication of validated models with any run-time parameters, files, sample data, baseline results, and metadata regarding the range of validity of the model. Such information would help to accelerate the use and improvement of the model.

The second function of the knowledge commons is to provide a collaborative environment for methods development, including access to the results of ruggedness testing and interlaboratory testing for a method, amplification regarding sample preparation and additional controls for different ENM types, and comments regarding modifications to improve reproducibility. Additional benefits for collaborative methods development include better understanding of the method, its range of validity, available instrumentation, and user facilities supporting the method. In addition, the knowledge commons would establish a means to publish, access, and annotate issues regarding analytic methods and their reproducibility.

The third function of the knowledge commons is to establish a means of collaboratively designing new ENMs by using models to encapsulate and quantify a material's characteristics and effects and potential risks associated with different manufacturing processes and controls. Because this function would provide useful results for manufacturers, regulators, and users of the materials, additional governance would be required to allow collaboration for precompetitive projects and continued use of modeling tools in a secure environment.

Although the knowledge commons would provide a new mechanism and environment for collaborative development of methods, models, and materials, many of the core functions have been initiated elsewhere. The Nanomaterial Registry (Nanomaterialregistry 2013) and NanoHUB (NanoHUB.org 2013) are two examples—the registry for sharing and annotating nanomaterial data and the NanoHUB for providing facilities for accessing, running, and annotating models. The underlying strength of the knowledge commons would be in linking these existing capabilities and others in a new environment focused on providing quantitative, reliable estimates of uncertainty for risk estimation and method validation and for establishing a vital missing link between the reductionist and integrative branches of research on the EHS aspects of nanotechnology. New programs, such as NanoRelease (ILSI 2013a) and NanoCharacter (ILSI 2013b), have similar aims, and the knowledge commons would aid in supporting government, industry, and academic participation in such programs. Such new initiatives as the Nanotechnology Knowledge Infrastructure (NSET 2012a; NNI 2013) and the Materials Genome Initiative (MGI) (NSTC 2011; EOP 2012; Warren and Boisvert 2012) could provide additional linkage and informatics expertise in augmenting the knowledge commons for different users and programs. Researchers involved in those initiatives are aware of each other's goals and progress because there is much overlap in membership, participation in each other's workshops, occasional briefings, and coordination through the National Nanotechnology Coordination Office (NNCO). However, discussions on an overarching framework that would knit their separate resources, capabilities, and objectives into the knowledge commons presented here have not yet taken place. Initiation of a series of pilots to integrate data and knowledge generated from the several activities and other informatics efforts would provide both a core planning group and an initial effort to set appropriate informatics requirements relevant to all activities whether private or public.

It is important to note that many other activities could provide valuable input into establishment of the knowledge commons and the present report is not intended to be comprehensive. Although this report is primarily focused on integrating research data, methods, and models relevant to the properties and effects of nanomaterials and nanomaterial-containing products in biologic and environmental systems, other related fields such as epidemiology and nanomedicine have not been the focus. However, the goals and structure of the knowledge commons are sufficiently broad to accommodate the integration of data, methods, and models used by stakeholders in these related fields. First, the evaluation of both EHS risk and product-design risk involves uncertainty propagation and the documentation and sharing of errors, uncertainties, sensitivities, and expert opinion through the knowledge commons and the informatics systems (see NRC 2012, pp.175-178 and Appendix B). Second, the emphasis on the need for data, method and model validation, curation, and sharing applies to all relevant fields, and reflects similar concerns and goals of other programs (for example, Big Data[1] and the MGI) as well as goals of the Network and Information Technology Research and Development (NITRD) program (NITRD 2013a). Third, as discussed in NRC 2012 (pp.175-178), existing nanoinformatics are compatible with National Cancer Institute and National Institutes of Health biomedical systems and applications, and recent progress, such as with the ISA-TAB-Nano data format capability extend that commonality to data exchange nomenclature and formats, including both genomics and clinical studies. Finally, there is evidence of convergence in vision among different informatics activities with examples, including US NanoHUB (NanoHUB.org 2013*)* and European Union NANOhub (JRC 2013), whose focus and goals overlap substantially, and collaborations involving EU-US CoRs and the NanoSafety Cluster (NanoSafety Cluster 2013).

Steps to Improve Progress in Developing the Knowledge Commons

Steps that could be taken to improve progress in development of the knowledge commons have been foreshadowed in the preceding pages and in Chapter 4 of the committee's first report (NRC 2012). The brief summary below broadly outlines the type of coordination that is needed to initiate development of a viable and vibrant knowledge commons that is responsive to the changing needs of the research and translational communities. The common theme under-

---

[1]For additional details see the workshop on Data Sharing and Metadata Curation: Obstacles and Strategies (NITRD 2013b).

lying model, method, and material development is the need to provide data and knowledge to improve the reproducibility of the models, methods, and materials.

To achieve reproducibility of models, there must be a means for publishing models with their run-time parameters, files, sample data, baseline results, and metadata concerning the range of validity. Virtual collaborative environments associated with each model or model type would allow focused scientific discussion of a particular model, its submodels, and algorithms; comparisons with similar models; and a means of establishing provenance concerning both model development and authorship. During model development (which accesses public data) the collaborative spaces should be open, permitting easy access for annotating and curating model development, the model's theoretical underpinnings, numerical methods and algorithms, and model validation. Access may be restricted for a number of reasons, but provision should be made for eventual publication of the model because scientific publication would be a primary motivator for placing it in the knowledge commons and would allow faster model improvement and adoption through an open-development infrastructure. As noted above, open development would be particularly suited to risk models in that modeling risk involves uncertainty propagation, whether the uncertainties arise from models, data, or expert opinion. Through use of the models to focus resources on reducing the largest uncertainties, the reproducibility of risk estimates could be improved systematically.

The use of virtual collaborative environments would also be key for methods development, creating a single focus for a method—its documentation and range of validity, accompanying video for adding detail or providing training, current instrumentation and later improvements, links to data obtained from the method and links to data and models derived from the data, annotation on the method and datasets, information on sample preparation and controls for different ENMs, and metadata and information regarding method curation and provenance. The primary advantages of the collaborative environments for analytic methods would be a common focus for all aspects of method development, robustness testing and capture of sensitivity data, interlaboratory testing and data capture, use of reference materials for calibration, suggestions for improvements and extensions, method revision and retesting, and provenance concerning all uses of the data. Standard methods could be developed, validated, adapted, improved, and revised on an abbreviated timescale while linkage to all raw, derived, and modeled data related to that method, its instrumentation, and sample preparation procedures is provided.

Virtual collaborative environments would also accelerate the development of nanomaterials. The collaborative environment could focus on a particular ENM designated by a production lot number; document the production, separation, and purification processes used and any initial characterization of the lot's properties; and create a data aggregation point for all uses of the particular nanomaterial, how samples were prepared, what methods were used, and whether the method's data were associated with any models or modeling efforts. Sample history could also be recorded; this would provide data necessary for both informal and formal interlaboratory testing of the materials with different methods. As data from different researchers using different methods are accumulated, comparisons can be made with greater validity because there would be a basis for "apple to apple"[2] comparisons, given the association among all samples that have common parentage. In addition, informed decisions concerning the structure or distribution of structures of particular ENM samples would be possible, and structural models of the samples could be deposited in a repository, such as the Collaboratory for Structural Nanobiology, for use in developing detailed predictive models of ENM effects in different environments. Collaboration spaces would also support aggregation of data on ENMs from different lots or from similar materials. Analysis of those data would allow correlation of ENM sample structures with their properties and effects and aid in formulating hypotheses of possible underlying mechanisms.

Perhaps the most important effect of the knowledge commons is the creation of a new literature based primarily on data from the application of validated methods to identified lots of nanomaterials. Raw data would be linked to derived data—whether on nanomaterial structure, their properties, or their effects in different experimental tests and environments—and to data from appropriate predictive and structural models. The correlation of data on ENM lot, structure, properties, and effects would help in the creation and incremental improvement of an evidence-based nomenclature and ontology that are consistent with known structural, experimental, and modeling data and that can be used to organize and track the use, annotation, curation, and provenance of the data and models in the knowledge commons. In addition, the informatics system could be implemented with different levels of security to accommodate both open exchanges with precompetitive data and models and privileged access for more restricted collaborative efforts.

NANOMATERIAL INTERACTIONS IN COMPLEX SYSTEMS RANGING FROM SUBCELLULAR SYSTEMS TO ECOSYSTEMS

As discussed in Chapter 3, the committee evaluated progress in a set of indicators related to ENM interactions in complex systems and found some progress. The indicators included extent of initiation of studies to relate in vitro to in vivo observations, extending research from simplified laboratory studies to more complex assays, and going from organisms to ecosystems; steps toward development of models for ecologic exposures and effects in complex systems; extent of refinement of a set of screening tools that reflect toxicity pathways; adapting existing system-level tools; and identification of benchmark or refer-

---

[2]The use of the phrase "apple to apple" comparisons conveys the importance of comparing sufficiently similar nanomaterials in studies (including such information as the material size, physical and chemical structure and properties, purity, and processes used to manufacture, store, and prepare the materials for analyses).

ence materials for use in development of tools for estimating exposures and doses and for providing positive and negative controls—useful for hazard ranking of ENMs. Perhaps one of the biggest gaps is the lack of mechanistic data—an increasing volume of toxicity data is being generated, but the ability to use the data to predict ENM risks with any certainty is constrained because of the types of studies conducted. Many of the published studies incorporate high-dose (overload) acute exposures to single cells or simplified single-organism mortality assays involving a single postexposure time and do not consider that underlying mechanisms are dose-dependent (Slikker et al. 2004). To provide more useful information, studies need to focus on more complex experimental design issues—such as relevant dose and dosimetry; dose response and time course characteristics; appropriate target cells, tissues, and organisms; and examination of more biologic pathways—concomitantly with better characterization of ENM test substances and incorporation of standardized reference materials as controls. The development and availability of standardized reference materials or benchmark (positive and negative) controls are essential because these materials are integral to study design. For example, use of ENM positive control material provides a reference for comparing the effects of ENM test materials being studied, and studies using ENM test materials and positive reference controls can facilitate comparisons of results among research laboratories, an essential component of the validation process.

In addition, consensus on the interpretation of hazard data is more readily achieved when the mechanism of action is known for the reference material. Useful comparisons are toxicity studies of endocrine disruption and 2,3,7,8-tetrachlorodibenzodioxin (TCDD); mechanisms are well known for the reference material (Eadon et al. 1986; Safe 1987, 1998; Van den Berg et al. 1998; Silva et al. 2002). Toxicity tests of potential estrogens or dioxins are done in reference to that of estrogen or TCDD and provide a comparison with the toxicity of the agent of interest, and they ensure that a study has a positive control. In contrast, for the development of validated assays for ENMs, no positive controls exist, partly because of the sparseness of information on potential mechanisms of action of ENMs. However, having available toxicologic data for ENMs once they have been more thoroughly studied, including an understanding of potential mechanisms, would help to advance the science. Thus, ENM reference and benchmark materials are needed for use by all researchers. A consistent set of reference and benchmark ENMs is also needed for each category, such as metal oxides, silver, gold, and carbon nanotubes (CNTs).

Additional shortcomings in available ENM toxicity data are related to the need to shift experimental study designs and models to gain more realistic and useful data for mechanistic understanding of ENMs. The preponderance of published studies provides information of questionable relevance to the health and environmental effects of realistic ENM exposures. Many findings are based on acute, high-dose exposures of single cells under in vitro conditions and so provide little or no information on relevant dose or dosimetry (for humans), on potential sustained effects (key to understanding potential toxicity vs short-term injury resulting from reactive oxidation species or an inflammatory response), on dose–response characteristics that provide mechanism insights, and on issues related to route of exposure or to life cycle. Similarly, many of the animal bioassay data come from studies involving high-dose acute exposures with limited time-course information or data on mechanisms or important end points, such as development and reproduction. In addition, there are minimal studies of community-level or ecosystem effects. Studies are limited to a few organisms, but uptake and mechanisms of action may differ among species. Those issues need to be explored further in relation to establishing standardized assays.

To generate study results that can provide useful information on potential health and environmental risks associated with ENMs and that can be validated by other researchers in the field, it will be important to expand and redirect the focus of experiments to provide greater relevance on EHS issues, considering the chronic low-dose exposure scenarios that prevail for people and ecosystems. The results should be shared with other investigators, and results of in vivo studies (at relevant concentrations) should be compared with results of in situ and in vitro screening assays to foster development of more expedient testing strategies. However, there is a paucity of useful in vivo data to establish a foundation for development of better screening tools. Consequently, the committee graded progress in experimental research in organisms that is relevant to community or ecosystem level effects as yellow. Research is ongoing in Environmental Protection Agency–National Science Foundation (EPA–NSF) centers, but there is little emphasis on the effects of ENM exposures on interactions among organisms (community-level effects) or on the interactions of multiple communities with the abiotic environment, including how ENMs may change such interactions and how ENMs may be changed when interacting within the ecosystem (ecosystem-level effects).

There is an absence of validated screening tools that are needed to apply data gained from experiments to challenging risk-related questions in humans and ecosystems (that is, transitioning from the laboratory world to the real world). There is a need to scale from laboratory systems to whole organisms and to the full ecosystem. Progress may need to be tied to a federal effort, inasmuch as individual laboratories may not have the incentive to participate in this methods development. One way to begin to address that shortcoming may be to use the data generated in the comprehensive Organisation for Economic Co-operation and Development program that involves 12 ENMs (representative of materials found in commerce). This program collects extensive in vivo health effects data in accordance with robust scientific guidelines (OECD 2013); the results could be used as benchmarks for toxicologic evaluation of unknown ENMs. New assays under development could be compared with that rich database. The lack of mechanistic understanding is a further barrier that limits certainty as to which types of assays should be developed. Supporting more mechanistic research and giving individual laboratories the opportunity to build on the few existing assays that have been tried with a subset of ENMs is necessary to bridge this gap.

Steps to Improve Progress in Understanding Nanomaterial Interactions in Complex Systems Ranging from Subcellular Systems to Ecosystems

The development of relevant in vivo hazard data based on appropriate routes of exposure and realistic exposure concentrations is an excellent starting point for understanding ENM interactions in complex systems. The ENM test material should be well characterized, and concentrations or doses administered to the organism should be based on data obtained from exposure-assessment studies and appropriate dose metrics (if available). Dose–response and time-course (temporal) characteristics should be built into the experimental design of these in vivo studies, and benchmark materials should be used as references for better interpretation of results. Time-course studies should initially focus on acute and subchronic responses to determine whether measurements of early (acute) injury are transitory. It would be important to have multiple laboratories conduct studies with similar or identical experimental protocols and end points to demonstrate whether interlaboratory experimental protocols and findings can be validated for a particular ENM or end point. When a more complete toxicologic profile of an ENM has been developed, in vitro models that use relevant cell types, end points, doses, and time-course results can be constructed. Well-designed, in vitro mechanistic studies can provide important insights into relevant toxicity pathways of a particular ENM response, but only when these criteria are established: there is a relevant in vivo end point for comparison, time-course studies are undertaken for both in vivo and in vitro investigations, appropriate doses and dose metrics are relevant for simulating human or ecologic exposures, temporal (time-course) effects are investigated (that is, not simply acute, high-dose effects), and appropriate benchmark reference materials are integrated into the experimental design to foster appropriate interpretation of the data. The successful establishment of adequate in vivo models should be followed sequentially by corresponding and validated in vitro toxicity tools; only then can the development of high-throughput toxicity screens informed by in situ and in vitro data represent a realistic approach.

ANALYSIS OF PROGRESS TOWARD ADDRESSING IMPLEMENTATION NEEDS

Indicators of Progress in Implementation and Their Link to the Nanotechnology Environmental, Health, and Safety Research Enterprise

The committee identified mechanisms to ensure implementation of the EHS research strategy, including enhancing interagency coordination, providing for stakeholder engagement in the research strategy, conducting and communicating results of research funded through public–private partnerships, and managing potential conflicts of interest (NRC 2012, p. 183). Each of those represents a high but achievable objective, and together they make up the support needed for implementation of a successful nanotechnology EHS research enterprise (Figure 4-1). For example, without strong and effective interagency coordination, a comprehensive knowledge commons is compromised. Robust interagency coordination minimizes overlap in research in the laboratory world and real world and maximizes the opportunity to identify research gaps and aggressively fund research needed to close them. Closing such gaps in turn supports the integration of all the elements in Figure 4-1; for example, with more and better data, modeling efforts can be improved, risk assessment can be enhanced, and decisions can be better informed.

Engagement of stakeholders in the research enterprise requires participation of all sectors, including government and academic researchers, nongovernment organizations (NGOs), regulators, industry, nanotechnology workers, and consumers. Stakeholder involvement maximizes the breadth of input needed to generate a comprehensive knowledge commons. Perhaps most important, stakeholders include workers and consumers who make up the populations that have the greatest exposures in the real world; these stakeholders not only have interest, expertise, and perspective in providing input that may help to shape research but are the most likely to be affected by the decisions made.

The role of public–private partnerships in the research portfolio for EHS aspects of ENMs has proved more difficult to define and implement. Funding and policy issues limit formation of such partnerships in that federal agencies involved in nanotechnology EHS research may have expended their allocated research budget and industry may have only modest interest in joint funding because of competitive business concerns. However, there are examples of successful public–private partnerships in the environmental-health arena. The most notable example has been the congressionally mandated Health Effects Institute (HEI), which operates through equal cofunding from EPA and the automobile industry. In the nanotechnology realm, examples include partnerships between the National Institute for Occupational Safety and Health (NIOSH) and industry, and the multistakeholder Nano Release Initiative, which provide collaboration and interaction beyond simply joint funding. Such partnerships can support focused research needs and could be well suited to develop inventories of ENMs and of their intended uses. Public–private partnerships also provide opportunities for development of instrumentation or methods to monitor or measure nanomaterial characteristics in laboratory and real-world research environments, which will enhance the knowledge commons. Well-structured and carefully governed public–private partnerships can provide unique credibility as they provide insulation against conflicts of interest.

The management of the potential for conflicts of interest between the dual roles of the National Nanotechnology Initiative (NNI) in both promoting and overseeing nanotechnology has special implications in Figure 4-1. Conflict of interest not only puts the knowledge commons at risk but has the potential to invalidate the models that are critical for assessing risk and supporting regulatory decisions. Management of conflict of interest can provide distinct lines of budget and management authority for applications-directed and implications-directed research. It can be facilitated by engaging a broad group of stakeholders with responsibility for helping to develop laboratory and real-world research. As noted previously, where feasible, appropriately structured public–private partnerships may offer unique opportunities for controlling and potentially eliminating conflict of interest in the data-collection process.

As described above and illustrated in Figure 4-1, all four implementation issues are central to the development of a successful nanotechnology EHS research enterprise. The discussion below addresses steps needed to "get to green" in the implementation indicators.

Steps to Ensure Progress Toward Enhancing Interagency Coordination

In Chapter 3, the committee recognizes the progress that the NNI has made in coordination of EHS research among federal agencies but reiterates the need for accountability for implementation of the NNI's EHS research strategy and the need for the strategy's integration with research undertaken by other entities, both domestically and internationally. The committee considers that little or no progress (red) has been made in "establishing a mechanism to ensure sufficient management and budgetary authority to implement the NNI's EHS research strategy" (NRC 2012, p. 183). However, it determined that some progress (yellow) had been made by the NNCO in annually identifying funding needs for interagency collaboration. Greater effort is needed specifically to accelerate and enhance high-priority research.

The need for a stronger, central convening authority to direct EHS research efforts conducted under the NNI has now been raised in at least four separate reviews of the NNI and its strategy (NRC 2009; GAO 2012; NRC 2012; PCAST 2012). As noted in Chapter 2, the latest President's Council of Advisors on Science and Technology (PCAST) review of the NNI identified "significant hurdles to an optimal structure and management" (p. 17), reiterating a concern that PCAST had raised in its 2010 review of the NNI (PCAST 2010): that NNI agency representatives on the Nanoscale Science, Engineering, and Technology Subcommittee (NSET) of the National Science and Technology Council Committee on Technology lack authority to influence budget allocations, even within their own agencies, that are needed to meet NNI objectives. In particular, PCAST called on the NSET to establish "high-level, cross-agency authoritative and accountable governance" (p. 22), noting that one effect of the absence of such a governance framework is a continuing gap between funded research and the information needed by decision-makers to manage potential risks effectively.

The present committee's first report (NRC 2012, pp. 166–169) proposed several options for establishing such authority, either inside or outside the NNI and the Nanotechnology Environmental Health Implications working group (NEHI) structure. Implementing those or other options need not require new legislation, but there may be advantages in pursuing such authority in any reauthorization of the 21st Century Nanotechnology Research and Development Act, as was considered but not enacted by the 111th Congress. Whatever the mechanism used, the committee reiterates the conclusion of its first report that "to implement [the NNI's] strategy effectively an entity with sufficient management and budgetary authority is needed to direct development and implementation of a federal EHS research strategy throughout NNI agencies and to ensure its integration with EHS research undertaken in the private sector, the academic community, and international organizations. Progress in implementation of the strategy will be severely limited in the absence of such an entity" (NRC 2012, p. 169).

Short of addressing that fundamental need, the committee suggested other means by which the NNI could enhance and extend interagency coordination. The NNI has identified a number of activities aimed at improving interagency coordination and stakeholder engagement, both in its 2011 EHS research strategy (NEHI 2011) and in its 2013 budget supplement (NSET 2012b), that are promising but do not appear to have been implemented. The 2011 strategy (NEHI 2011, p. 96) indicates plans to use "webinars, workshops, and other mechanisms for information exchange to assess the state of the science and current research, and to reassess areas of weakness and gaps"; however, despite proposing to host two or three webinars each year, it appears that the NNI has held but one such webinar, "Public Engagement through Nano.gov" (NNI 2012a), and at the time of this writing none is planned.

The NNI's 2011 strategy also identified its signature initiatives (NNI 2012b) as offering NEHI "a new mechanism through which to organize and leverage interagency efforts" (NEHI 2011, p. 96). Those initiatives are all focused on nanotechnology development, however, not on EHS issues, and the committee has not seen any indications of NEHI's use of the signature initiatives for the indicated purpose. Similarly, the NNI's 2013 budget supplement (NSET 2012b, p. 61) notes plans for NEHI to host "monthly meetings, public workshops and webinars and other social media", but the committee is not aware that such activities have taken place. The committee encourages NEHI and the NNCO to implement those plans, which promise the dual benefit of enhancing interagency coordination and stakeholder engagement.

Another option would be the formal assignment of responsibility for management of the knowledge commons shown in Figure 4-1 to the NNCO. The NNCO would then be accountable for ensuring both that EHS-relevant information generated by research in individual NNI agencies is efficiently transferred to the knowledge commons and that it is widely shared. Such responsibility in itself might support and spur a greater role for the NNCO in enhancing interagency coordination. The committee puts this example forth to illustrate the role that enhanced interagency coordination could play in increasing the overall effectiveness and efficiency of the nanotechnology EHS research enterprise.

At the committee's November 2012 workshop, representatives of two federal agencies indicated that they were undertaking a mapping of their own research activities onto the 2011 NNI strategy's objectives. The NNCO could require all NNI agencies to conduct such mapping, compile the results, and use them to indicate how they intend to address overlaps and gaps in their activities.

Finally, to address PCAST's criticism directly, the NNCO could reconstitute the NSET to require that NNI agencies designate senior officials who have budgetary authority in their agencies as members of the NSET.

Improving interagency coordination requires tracking of research that is being conducted by the agencies and of how much is being spent on specific projects. Since publication of the committee's first report, two reviews of the NNI have raised concerns about the need for the NNI to develop and implement better performance metrics that can be used to track progress toward core objectives. That need was a central theme of the 2012 Government Accountability Office (GAO) report, which has as one of its two "recommendations for executive action" that "the Director of OSTP [Office of Science and Technlogy Policy] coordinate development by the NNI member agencies of performance measures, targets, and time frames for nanotechnology EHS research that align with the research needs of the NNI, consistent with the agencies' respective statutory authorities, and include this information in publicly available reports" (p. 51). GAO (2012, p. 46) noted that earlier reviews had also flagged that need, including a 2010 review by the National Nanotechnology Advisory Panel (PCAST 2010) and NRC (2009).

Similarly, PCAST's 2012 review of the NNI (pp. vi, 17) notes that "the lack of clear metrics for assessing the impacts of Federal investments in nanotechnology remains a concern" and that it had raised a similar concern in its 2010 review of the NNI. PCAST calls on agencies to develop "mission-appropriate" (p. 21) metrics and on the NNCO to track the development of appropriate metrics and implement them to assess NNI outputs. (PCAST's call for such metrics is not limited to EHS concerns; it is related to all aspects of the NNI.)

Metrics are needed specifically for identifying the levels, types, and sources of funding needed to ensure that interagency research efforts have sufficient funding to meet specific goals and to complete research in fields identified as having high priority.[3] As noted earlier, the committee continues to believe that accountability for fostering interagency collaboration in implementing a research strategy requires more than what the NNI has done to date—identifying what collaborative research is under way or contemplated—namely, putting into place a means of estimating periodically (ideally at least once a year) funding needs and of tracking and reporting progress toward meeting the needs. GAO (2012, p. 51) reached a similar conclusion: "We also recommend that, to the extent possible, the Director of OSTP coordinate the development by the NNI member agencies of estimates of the costs and types of resources necessary to meet the EHS research needs."

---

[3]The absence of available funding data prevented the committee from revisiting the resource estimates presented in its first report (NRC 2012).

The committee is not aware of any effort by the NNCO to develop such a set of metrics for estimating funding needs and tracking whether they are met. We renew our call for the NNCO to do so.

Steps to Ensure Progress Toward Addressing Stakeholder Involvement

In Chapter 3, the committee rated progress toward "actively engaging diverse stakeholders in a continuing manner" (NRC 2012, p. 183) as yellow and noted some specific examples of progress toward meeting this goal. Getting to green in stakeholder engagement means encouraging the bright spots where there is some momentum, simultaneously expanding on existing programs and creating new ones. The NIOSH forum (NIOSH 2012) should be supported as an annual event, not where the research and development (R&D) community is located but where the opportunity for the greatest stakeholder engagement can be found, and should be marketed directly to the stakeholder groups that were underrepresented in the "first annual" event. Similar forums should be created, perhaps aligned with the EHS categories of worker–consumer–environment or value chain (raw materials–intermediates–final products). The forums could be extended into standing bodies to ensure that stakeholder-engagement processes are ongoing and inform all aspects of strategy development, implementation, and revision. The public forums and standing bodies are critical for generating and building engagement among the various stakeholders and will lead to more buy-in at the outset of and throughout these processes.

In addition, the committee recommends the creation of a new Stakeholder Advisory Council by the NNCO. It would help the NNCO to assess the effectiveness of such efforts as those described in the previous paragraph and identify opportunities to expand such forums to include other stakeholder groups and all aspects of the research strategy. The members of the Stakeholder Advisory Council would become key points of contact for the stakeholders that they represent that might be underserved, marketing such programs directly to their peers, and collecting responses from them regarding better ways to engage.

There are models for such an advisory council. In its 2012 report (NRC 2012, pp. 170-171), the committee described NIOSH's National Occupational Research Agenda (NORA), specifically its establishment of both sector-specific councils and a cross-sector council. Council members assist the institute in developing, implementing, and revising national and sector research agendas and strategies, and in facilitating communications to and from their respective stakeholder groups. The Stakeholder Advisory Council of Australia's National Enabling Technologies Strategy offers another model (Australian Government 2013). This standing council with diverse stakeholder representation meets regularly to advise the government on nanotechnology and other enabling technologies. Its focus is broader than NORA but includes research strategies, including policy issues, funding needs and priorities, sector and community communications and engagement, and information dissemination.

Steps to Ensure Progress Toward Development of Public–Private Partnerships

The committee determined that little or no progress had been made in creating well-defined effective partnerships as measured by execution of partnership agreements, issuance of requests for proposals, and the establishment of governance structure—hence, it denoted this indicator as red. Although there have been few nanotechnology-based public–private partnerships, blueprints from other scientific fields exist, such as the HEI. Founded in 1980, the HEI is a nonprofit corporation chartered to provide scientific research on the health effects of air pollution. Its mission is to identify and fund high-priority research, to provide independent review of HEI-based research, and to communicate HEI's results.

The HEI has funded and published or presented public reports on more than 250 studies on a variety of topics, including carbon monoxide, air toxics, nitrogen oxides, diesel exhaust, ozone, particulate matter, and other pollutants. Its board of directors includes leaders of corporations, academe, NGOs, and policy groups. EPA and representatives from the motor-vehicle industry—Ford Motor Company, General Motors Corporation, and Chrysler LLC—fund the organization, each with about a 50% share.

In addition to NIOSH's nanotechnology-focused public–private partnerships discussed in Chapter 3, a nanotechnology EHS–focused public–private partnership that could serve as a model was the Europe-based Nanotechnology Capacity Building NGOs (NanoCap) (NanoCap 2009). The European Commission, under the FP6 Science and Society programme, funded the 3-year project (2006–2009) which was organized to increase understanding of EHS risks and ethical aspects of nanotechnology. IVAM is an independent research and consulting firm of the University of Amsterdam Holding in the Netherlands that conducts technologic, environmental, and occupational-health projects with trade unions, environmental NGOs, industry, and government organizations. It led a consortium of environmental NGOs (for example, the Baltic Environmental Forum, the European Environmental Bureau, and the Mediterranean Information Office for Environment, Culture and Sustainable Development), trade unions (such as European Trade Union Institute, Health and Safety Department), and academic researchers (such as at the University of Aarhus interdisciplinary Nanoscience center, Katholieke Universiteit Leuven, the Department of Public health, the University of Amsterdam, and the Institute for Biodiversity and Ecosystem Dynamics). NanoCap developed and publically presented recommendations that enabled public authorities to address EHS risks related to nanotechnology. In addition, NanoCap's goal was to encourage academe and industry to focus on reduction of sources of nanoparticles and the inclusion of risk assessment in their work.

The NNI signature initiatives are additional examples of public–private partnerships, albeit not focused on EHS. The signature initiatives are collaborations intended to spur the advancement of nanotechnology in the service of national economic, security, and environmental goals. For example, the signature initiative Nanotechnology Knowledge Infrastructure: Enabling National Leadership in Sustainable Design is a multistakeholder group of scientists, engineers, and federal agencies charged with developing a multidisciplinary collaboration that integrates basic research, modeling, applications development, and ultimately a nanotechnology data infrastructure to support data-sharing and collaboration (NNI 2013).

Overall, getting to green on "conducting and communicating the results of research funded through public–private partnerships" may require a public–private partnership approach similar to the HEI but with a focus on nanotechnology EHS issues, such as NIOSH's efforts or the European-based NanoCap. Five critical elements for an effective public–private partnership are a strong independent and accountable governance structure, adequate and shared funding, specific and agreed-on goals, transparent sharing of results and information, and appropriate confidentiality agreements. To that end, the committee recommends that NNI government agencies, individually and jointly, spur the organization of well-focused public–private partnerships; however, the governance structure needs to extend well beyond the agency. For example, HEI's Board of Directors is a recommended governance model. However, unlike the HEI's automotive-industry focus, no single market or industry binds all nanotechnology research, so there may be a need to establish multiple sector-specific or material-based public–private partnerships (for example, a CNT-based public–private partnership that includes CNT manufacturers, researchers, and other key stakeholders).

Partners should share in the funding of the public–private partnerships; this would help to ensure active participation of all parties in moving toward clearly articulated and agreed-on goals. Although the goals will depend on the nature and scope of the specific partnership, some basic goals modeled on those of HEI would provide direction applicable to all public–private partnerships.

Public–private partnerships should foster open sharing of information, both internally among partners and externally with a broader audience, via reports, conferences, and other media. Public–private partnership agreements should take into account the confidentiality concerns of industrial partners. It is understood that the organization of an effective and well-run public–private partnership takes time, but NNI agencies should increase their efforts to initiate partnership programs because they are critical for the implementation of the research strategy; without them, research progress will be slower and more limited.

The committee recognizes that there are mechanisms that allow agencies to share and pool resources for collaborative projects. An example is the joint funding of federally funded research and development centers (FFRDCs), such as the EPA- and NSF-funded University of California Center for Environmental Implications of Nanotechnology and the Center for Environmental Implications of Nanotechnology.

Steps to Ensure Progress Toward Addressing Conflict of interests

Conflict of interest is an issue of public concern that affects many societal sectors and institutions, both public and private. From government agencies, academic institutions, and professional organizations to industry, financial institutions, and nonprofit organizations, that concern has resulted in the proliferation of conflict-of-interest policies, reporting and disclosure requirements, and training programs meant to restore or ensure public confidence and trust.

In one widely used definition, conflict of interest is described as "a set of circumstances that creates a risk that professional judgment or actions regarding a primary interest will be unduly influenced by a secondary interest" (Lo and Field 2009, p. 46). By statute, the NNI was established with dual functions—promoting the development and commercialization of nanotechnology applications and understanding and mitigating their EHS implications—and that created a set of circumstances in which conflict of interest is almost inherent.

The current allocation of its research dollars ($105 million requested for EHS research in 2013 of a total NNI request of $1.8 billion) is perhaps the most visible manifestation of the conflict. It is clear that applications R&D takes priority over EHS risk research, so it is understandable that some stakeholders may question or have concerns about the NNI's ability to pursue research on EHS implications with vigor and integrity. The tension between the dual roles of NNI is exacerbated in that the results of EHS research may inform regulatory decisions and affect the developers and users of nanotechnology applications.

Given the almost inherent conflict, it is critical that the NNI focus particular attention and energy on ensuring that all stakeholders—including workers and the consuming public—trust the integrity of its EHS research enterprise. As noted in the committee's first report, the separation of nuclear-power R&D (assigned to the Department of Energy) from risk research and risk management (assigned to the Nuclear Regulatory Commission) is one model for addressing the inherent conflict between the federal government's interest in developing a new technology and managing the associated risks.

In Chapter 3, the committee assessed progress toward addressing two indicators for managing conflicts of interest. The committee determined that little progress had been made toward "achieving a clear separation in management and budgetary authority and accountability between the functions of developing and promoting applications of nanotechnology and understanding and assessing its potential health and environmental implications" (NRC 2012, p. 183), and this indicator was designated red. Some progress was deemed to have been made in the "continued separate tracking and reporting of EHS research activities and funding" (NRC 2012, p. 183), so this indicator was yellow.

To move those indicators toward green, actual or perceived conflicts that arise from the NNI's dual mission could be addressed through structural and managerial changes—driven by changes in the NNI's authorizing statute or by changes that the NNI and its participating agencies could implement themselves. Such changes do not seem to be forthcoming; indeed, in its 2013 budget supplement (NSET 2012b), the NNI noted that such actions are "unlikely or not needed". The committee continues to believe that the NNI writ large would benefit from a clearer separation of authority and accountability for its EHS research enterprise. It would not only advance stakeholder trust and confidence in the seriousness of the NNI's commitment to responsible development, especially the integral importance of its EHS research mission, but would help to address the need for better integration and coordination of EHS research throughout the NNI. The committee urges the NNI to review and reconsider the variety of models, mechanisms, and managerial processes noted in the committee's first report. Until such changes in structure, management, and budgetary processes are made, greater transparency will be key in getting to green.

Even within its current remit, greater transparency can help to address concerns about possible conflicts of interest and real or perceived bias within the NNI research community.[4] The NNI has already made some progress in enhancing transparency for its EHS research, for example, by improving the tracking and reporting of EHS research activities and funding and by providing narrative information on agency-specific EHS research activities and projects in the NNI supplement to the president's FY 2013 budget. Further efforts to enhance the timeliness, specificity, and accessibility of information about EHS research projects are needed, including development of clearer guidance on how agencies should differentiate between research directly relevant to EHS risk and applications-oriented research with EHS implications.

Transparency and trust can be further advanced through creation of and adherence to strong scientific-integrity policies at the agency level. Following a presidential memo on the topic, OSTP issued guidelines for scientific-integrity policies in 2010 (Holdren 2010), and most departments have developed policies and plans in response.[5] The NNI should periodically review the scientific-integrity policies of its participating agencies to ensure continued attention and adherence to the key principles of scientific integrity—a cornerstone of public trust in the scientific enterprise of public agencies.

The NSET, the NNCO, and NNI agencies should explore additional mechanisms to foster transparency and thus minimize and manage any concerns about conflicts of interest and bias. For example, the NNCO or NNI agencies could create an ombudsman position to receive, investigate, and resolve complaints or concerns about bias and conflicts of interest in the NNI's research portfolio. The NNCO could also develop and disseminate best practices for

---

[4]For definitions of conflict of interest and bias, see Appendix B in the Keystone Center's report from the Research Integrity Roundtable, *Improving the Use of Science in Regulatory Decision-making: Dealing with Conflict of Interest and Bias in Scientific Advisory Panels and Improving Systematic Scientific Reviews* (Keystone Center 2012). For hypothetical examples of conflict of interest and bias, see Appendix 1 in the Bipartisan Policy Center report *Improving the Use of Science in Regulatory Policy* (Bipartisan Policy Center 2009).

[5]For an assessment of and link to agency scientific-integrity policies, see UCS (2012).

identifying, managing, and preventing conflicts of interest and bias in the planning, conduct, and reporting of research—especially for entities engaged in research on both nanoscience applications and their EHS implications. Identification of best practices, with appropriate checks and balances, should be informed by input provided through a multistakeholder process that includes workers, consumers, health and environmental NGOs, large and small businesses, and researchers in the public and private sectors. Attention to frequency, timeliness, substance, and inclusivity of stakeholder engagement activities can also enhance trust and transparency.

REFERENCES

Australian Government. 2013. National Enabling Technologies Strategy: A National Approach. Department of Industry, Innovation, Climate Change, Science, Research and Tertiary Education [online]. Available: http://www.innovation.gov.au/ Industry/Nanotechnology/NationalEnablingTechnologiesStrategy/Pages/National EnablingTechnologiesStrategyANationalApproach.aspx [accessed June 20, 2013].

Badireddy, A.R., M.R. Wiesner, and J. Liu. 2012. Detection, characterization, and abundance of engineered nanoparticles in complex waters by hyperspectral imagery with enhanced darkfield microscopy. Environ. Sci. Technol. 46(18):10081-10088.

Bipartisan Policy Center. 2009. Improving the Use of Science in Regulatory Policy. Science for Policy Project [online]. Available: http://bipartisanpolicy.org/sites/default/ files/BPC%20Science%20Report%20fnl.pdf [accessed Dec. 27, 2012].

Eadon, G., L. Kaminsky, J. Silkworth, K. Aldous, D. Hilker, P. O'Keefe, R. Smith, J. Gierthy, J. Hawley, N. Kim, and A. DeCaprio. 1986. Calculation of 2, 3, 7, 8-TCDD equivalent concentrations of complex environmental contaminant mixtures. Environ. Health Perspect. 70:221-227.

EOP (Executive Office of the President). 2012. Fact Sheet: Progress on Materials Genome Initiative, May 14, 2012. Executive Office of the President [online]. Available: http://www.whitehouse.gov/sites/default/files/microsites/ostp/mgi_fact_sheet_ 05_14_2012_final.pdf [accessed Mar. 12, 2013].

GAO (U.S. Government Accountability Office). 2012. Nanotechnology: Improved Performance Information Needed for Environmental, Health, and Safety Research. GAO-12-427. Washington, DC: U.S. Government Accountability Office [online]. Available: http://www.gao.gov/assets/600/591007.pdf [accessed Dec. 5, 2012].

Holdren, J.P. 2010. Scientific Integrity. Memorandum for the Heads of Executive Departments and Agencies, from John P. Holdren, Assistant to the President for Science and Technology and Director of the Office of Science and Technology, Washington, DC. December 17, 2010 [online]. Available: http://www.whitehouse.gov/sites/de fault/files/microsites/ostp/scientific-integrity-memo-12172010.pdf [accessed Apr. 8, 2013].

Hou, W.C., P. Westerhoff, and J.D. Posner. 2013. Biological accumulation of engineered nanomaterials: A review of current knowledge. Environ. Sci. Process. Impacts 15(1): 103-122.

ILSI (International Life Sciences Institute). 2013a. NanoRelease Consumer Products [online]. Available: http://www.ilsi.org/ResearchFoundation/RSIA/Pages/NanoRel ease1.aspx [accessed Mar. 12, 2013].

ILSI (International Life Science Institute). 2013b. NanoCharacter [online]. Available: http://www.ilsi.org/NanoCharacter/Pages/NanoCharacter.aspx [accessed Mar. 12, 2013].

JRC (Joint Research Centre Institute). 2013. JRCNANOhub. European Commission, Joint Research Centre Institute, Institute for Health and Consumer Protection (IHCP), Ispra [online]. Available: http://www.napira.eu/ [accessed Mar. 12, 2013].

Keystone Center. 2012. Improving the Use of Science in Regulatory Decision-Making: Dealing with Conflict of Interest and Bias in Scientific Advisory Panels, and Improving Systematic Scientific Reviews. A Report from the Research Integrity Roundtable [online]. Available: https://www.keystone.org/images/keystone-center/spp-documents/Health/Research%20Integrity%20Rountable%20Report.pdf [accessed Dec. 27, 2012].

Lo, B., and M.J. Field, eds. 2009. Conflict of Interest in Medical Research, Education, and Practice. Washington, DC: National Academies Press.

Lombi, E., E. Donner, E. Tavakkoli, T.W. Turney, R. Naidu, B.W. Miller, and K.G. Scheckel. 2012. Fate of zinc oxide nanoparticles during anaerobic digestion of wastewater and post-treatment processing of sewage sludge. Environ. Sci. Technol. 46(16):9089-9096.

Mitrano, D.M., A. Barber, A. Bednar, P. Westerhoff, C.P. Higgins, and J.F. Ranville. 2012. Silver nanoparticle characterization using single particle ICP-MS (SP-ICP-MS) and asymmetrical flow field flow fractionation ICP-MS (AF4-ICP-MS). J. Anal. At. Spectrom. 27(7):1131-1142.

NanoCap. 2009. NanoCap Project. European FP6 Capacity Building Project [online]. Available: http://www.nanocap.eu/Flex/Site/Page4662.html?PageID=%26Lang= [accessed Apr.8, 2013].

NanoHUB.org. 2013. NanoHUB [online]. Available: http://nanohub.org/ [accessed Mar. 12, 2013].

Nanomaterialregistry.org. 2013. Nanomaterial Registry [online]. Available: https://www.nanomaterialregistry.org/ [accessed Mar. 12, 2013].

NanoSafety Cluster. 2013. About NanoSafety Cluster [online]. Available: http://www.nanosafetycluster.eu/ [accessed July 11, 2013].

NEHI (Nanotechnology Environmental Health Implications Working Group). 2011. National Nanotechnology Initiative 2011 Environmental, Health, and Safety Strategy, October 2011. Nanotechnology Environmental Health Implications Working Group, Subcommittee on Nanoscale Science, Engineering, and Technology, Committee on Technology, National Science and Technology Council [online]. Available: http://www.nano.gov/sites/default/files/pub_resource/nni_2011_ehs_research_strategy.pdf [accessed Dec. 27, 2012].

NIOSH (National Institute for Occupational Safety and Health). 2012. Prevention through Design: Safe Nano Design Workshop, August 14-16, 2012, Albany, NY [online]. Available: http://www.cdc.gov/niosh/topics/ptd/nanoworkshop/default.html [accessed Feb. 2, 2013].

NITRD (The Networking and Information Technology Research and Development). 2013a. Networking and Information Technology Research and Development Program, NITRD Subcommittee [online]. Available: http://www.nitrd.gov/nitrdgroups/index.php?title=Subcommittee_on_Networking_and_Information_Technology_Research_and_Development_(NITRD_Subcommittee) [accessed July 12, 2013].

NITRD (The Networking and Information Technology Research and Development). 2013b. Data Sharing and Metadata Curation: Obstacles and Strategies: Future Strategies for Managing Scientific Data and Metadata for Basic and Applied Research, May 29, 2013, Natural Science Foundation, Arlington, VA [online]. Available: http://www.nitrd.gov/nitrdgroups/index.php?title=Data_Sharing_and_Meta data_Curation:_Obstacles_and_Strategies [accessed July 12, 2013].

NNI (U.S. National Nanotechnology Initiative). 2012a. Public Engagement through Nano.gov. Webinar. Nano.gov [online]. Available: http://www.nano.gov/node/873 [accessed Dec. 27, 2012].

NNI (U.S. National Nanotechnology Initiative). 2012b. Nanotechnology Signature Initiatives. Nano.gov. [online]. Available: http://www.nano.gov/signatureinitiatives [accessed Dec. 27, 2012].

NNI (U.S. National Nanotechnology Initiative). 2013. NSI: Nanotechnology Knowledge Initiative (NKI) – Enabling National Leadership in Sustainable Design [online]. Available: http://www.nano.gov/node/829 [accessed Mar. 12, 2013].

NRC (National Research Council). 2009. Review of the Federal Strategy for Nanotechnology-Related Environmental, Health, and Safety Research. Washington, DC: National Academies Press.

NRC (National Research Council). 2011. Toward Precision Medicine: Building a Knowledge Network for Biomedical Research and a New Taxonomy of Disease. Washington, DC: National Academies Press.

NRC (National Research Council). 2012. A Research Strategy for Environmental, Health, and Safety Aspects of Engineered Nanomaterials. Washington, DC: National Academies Press.

NSET (Nanoscale Science, Engineering, and Technology). 2012a. Nanotechnology Signature Initiative. Nanotechnology Knowledge Infrastructure: Enabling National Leadership in Sustainable Design. Subcommittee on Nanoscale Science, Engineering, and Technology, National Science and Technology Council. May 14, 2012 [online]. Available: http://nano.gov/sites/default/files/pub_resource/nki_nsi_white_paper_-_final_for_web.pdf [accessed Jan. 22, 2013].

NSET (Nanoscale Science, Engineering, and Technology Subcommittee). 2012b. The National Nanotechnology Initiative: Research and Development Leading to a Revolution in Technology and Industry: Supplement to the President's FY 2013 Budget. Subcommittee on Nanoscale Science, Engineering, and Technology, National Science and Technology Council. February 2012 [online]. Available: http://www.nano.gov/sites/default/files/pub_resource/nni_2013_budget_supplement.pdf [accessed Nov. 27, 2012].

NSTC (National Science Technology Council). 2011. Materials Genome Initiative for Global Competitiveness. Interagency Group on Advanced Materials, National Science Technology Council. June 2011 [online]. Available: http://nano.gov/node/829 [accessed Mar. 12, 2013].

OECD (Organisation for Economic Co-operation and Development). 2013. Current Developments in Delegations on the Safety of Manufactured Nanomaterials – Tour de Table. Series on the Safety of Manufactured Nanomaterials No. 37. ENV/JM/MONO (2013)2. Organisation for Economic Co-operation and Development [online]. Available: http://search.oecd.org/officialdocuments/displaydocumentpdf/?cote=env/jm/mono%282013%292&doclanguage=en [accessed Mar. 11, 2013].

PCAST (President's Council of Advisors on Science and Technology). 2010. Report to the President and Congress on the Third Assessment of the National Nanotechnology Initiative. March 2010 [online]. Available: http://www.whitehouse.gov/sites/default/files/microsites/ostp/pcast-nano-report.pdf [accessed Dec. 20, 2012].

PCAST (President's Council of Advisors on Science and Technology). 2012. Report to the President and Congress on the Fourth Assessment of the National Nanotechnology Initiative. April 2012 [online]. Available: http://nano.gov/sites/default/files/pub_resource/pcast_2012_nanotechnology_final.pdf [accessed Dec. 5, 2010].

Safe, S. 1987. Determination of 2,3,7,8-TCDD toxic equivalent factors (TEFs): Support for the use of the in vitro AHH induction assay. Chemosphere 16(4):791-802.

Safe, S.H. 1998. Hazard and risk assessment of chemical mixtures using the toxic equivalency factor approach. Environ. Health Perspect. 106(suppl. 4):1051-1058.

Silva, E., N. Rajapakse, and A. Kortenkamp. 2002. Something from "nothing": Eight weak estrogenic chemicals combined at concentrations below NOECs produce significant mixture effects. Environ. Sci. Technol. 36(8):1751-1756.

Slikker, W., Jr., M.E. Andersen, M.S. Bogdanffy, J.S. Bus, S.D. Cohen, R.B. Conolly, R.M. David, N.G. Doerrer, D.C. Dorman, D.W. Gaylor, D. Hattis, J.M. Rogers, R.W. Setzer, J.A. Swenberg, and K. Wallace. 2004. Dose-dependent transitions in mechanisms of toxicity: Case studies. Toxicol. Appl. Pharmacol. 201(3):226-294.

UCS (Union of Concerned Scientists). 2012. Agency-specific Solutions. Union of Concerned Scientists, Cambridge, MA [online]. Available: http://staff.nationalacademies.org/academynet/informationresources/researchcenter/index.htm [accessed Apr. 8, 2013].

Van den Berg, M., L. Birnbaum, A.T. Bosveld, B. Brunström, P. Cook, M. Feeley, J.P. Giesy, A. Hanberg, R. Hasegawa, S.W. Kennedy, T. Kubiak, J.C. Larsen, F.X. van Leeuwen, A.K. Liem, C. Nolt, R.E. Peterson, L. Poellinger, S. Safe, D. Schrenk, D. Tillitt, M. Tysklind, M. Younes, F. Waern, and T. Zacharewski. 1998. Toxic equivalency factors (TEFs) for PCBs, PCDDs, PCDFs for humans and wildlife. Environ. Health Perspect. 106(12):775-792.

Warren, J.A., and R.F. Boisvert. 2012. Building the Materials Innovation Infrastructure: Data and Standards. A Materials Genome Initiative Workshop, May15-15, 2012, Washington, DC. NISTIR 7898. National Institute of Standards and Technology [online]. Available: http://nvlpubs.nist.gov/nistpubs/ir/2012/NIST.IR.7898.pdf [accessed Apr. 5, 2013].

Westerhoff, P., and B. Nowack. 2013. Searching for global descriptors of engineered nanomaterial fate and transport in the environment. Acc. Chem. Res. 46(3):844-853.

5

Going Beyond Green

INTRODUCTION: A VISION FOR THE FUTURE

In the previous chapters of this report, the committee examined research and infrastructure developments related to environmental, health, and safety (EHS) aspects of engineered nanomaterials (ENMs). The committee assessed findings from recently released US and European Union reports that provide global perspectives on the needs for advancing EHS nanotechnology research (see discussion in Chapter 2). The committee examined trajectories of progress in the research and infrastructure priorities articulated in its first report (Chapter 3) and identified critical barriers to progress and steps that are needed to ensure that progress is made (that is, to get to green) (Chapter 4). The present chapter builds on Chapters 3 and 4 to address overarching issues that are relevant to ensuring timely progress in the committee's research priorities. It amplifies issues included in the overall charge on the basis of the committee's review of progress since the first report and provides a means to address the criteria for assessing research progress over the longer-term described in that first report. As part of this evaluation, the committee presents a construct (Figure 4-1) that provides an overall vision of a comprehensive research enterprise on the potential EHS risks posed by ENMs, capturing the interrelated and interdependent research activities that are driven by the evolving production of ENMs. That construct highlights critical interactions among members of the research community and the wider group of stakeholders and the importance of a coordinated infrastructure to ensure that the efforts of the research community are optimized. These themes are reflected in the committee's longer-term criteria for addressing research progress and address issues such as the level of interaction and collaboration among key stakeholders; the coordination and integration of the research strategy with regards to planning, budgeting, and management; accessibility of information to interested stakeholders; and the feasibility of conducting the research in a timely manner so that it is responsive to stakeholder and decision-maker needs.

In this chapter, the committee provides a broader perspective and suggestions for creating a successful portfolio of risk-related research. Both here and in the first report, the committee has highlighted that *how* a research strategy is implemented is just as central to its success as is its scientific or technical content. A strategy for risk research should recognize the inherent technical and cultural obstacles that researchers and the broader community can face in building knowledge about potential EHS risks. Such considerations are vital for creating a robust global research community that can successfully identify the risks associated with emerging ENMs while providing strategies for minimizing the risks. A successful research enterprise, as shown in Figure 4-1, will provide findings of immediate relevance to the responsible development of nanotechnology, and sustaining that enterprise will be of interest to all its diverse stakeholders to ensure that risk is effectively managed.

This chapter offers a vision of a global research enterprise that will be the vehicle for answering current and future questions about the potential risks posed to human health and the environment by ENMs. The overarching (or ultimate) goal of the enterprise is to generate the information needed to design materials and processes to be safer from the outset—to reduce or eliminate hazards and risks to human health and the environment; for example, see Hutchison (2008) on "greener nanoscience" and NIOSH (2012) for a more general description of "prevention through design". In this chapter, the committee projects to a time beyond the domain of its current research recommendations to consider how questions about risk can be best approached in an adaptive and continuing manner so as to update priorities for research and identify concerns constantly. The chapter is aspirational and goes beyond setting out a prospective research portfolio to consider how future concerns can be anticipated and addressed.

The general approach recommended by this committee is germane not only to ENMs but more broadly to any emergent technology or class of materials that may be perceived to pose a risk. Prospective and continuing assessment of potential hazard clearly is vital, and Figure 4-1 incorporates three key elements of the approach that are the focus of this chapter and are discussed below:

- A **governance structure,** including designation of an institutional lead with sufficient authority and accountability, clearly defined metrics for gauging research progress, coordinated communications with and engagement of all stakeholders, leveraged public–private partnerships, and principles that prevent conflicts between applications and implications of nanotechnology research.
- **Stable, long-term support and incentives** for sustaining the research community and engaging interdisciplinary and international researchers.
- An **adaptive decision-making process** that integrates the latest nanotechnology EHS information from all over the world into a "knowledge commons" and provides sufficient funding and incentives, with input from multiple stakeholders, to illuminate the path toward ENM design, application, and high-priority risk research.

EFFECTIVE GOVERNANCE

Throughout its deliberations, the committee has repeatedly concluded that stronger governance of nanotechnology EHS research is needed to manage, direct, and disseminate results of the numerous research activities. Achieving effective governance is no small task. Considering the applications and implications of nanotechnology requires enormous scale, input from diverse sectors, and a comprehensive systems-driven approach to science. Unlike some other "big science" research approaches, such as the Human Genome Project, the applications of nanotechnology permeate virtually every sector of our society and economy. Such broad reach means that nanotechnology and related EHS issues span the missions and jurisdictions of many government agencies and intersect with the activities and interests of many stakeholders, including businesses, the academic community, consumers, workers, and myriad organizations that make up civil society. Governance should actively engage all those in the process of managing nanotechnology EHS research.

Nanotechnology's applications and its EHS implications are closely intertwined. That is, the novel or enhanced physical and chemical characteristics of ENMs (such as greater reactivity or solubility than that of the larger "bulk" material of the same chemical composition) that are being exploited in new applications may also lead to biologic behaviors of potential concern for environmental or human health. In addition, knowledge of the uncertainties in physical and chemical ENM characteristics is needed for estimation of design risk in the cases of materials, products, and applications and for estimation of EHS risks. Applications research is often relevant to our understanding of potential EHS risks and vice versa, and this highlights the need for close collaboration of researchers in both fields and for an infrastructure that supports more efficient and facile information flow between and integration of the applications-research and implications-research communities.

However, close researcher interaction does not necessarily imply that applications research and implications research should be jointly managed. Many agencies conduct or fund both applications research and implications research in nanotechnology under the aegis of the National Nanotechnology Initiative (NNI). That coordinating body has as its mission both the development of nanotechnology and ensuring that such development is socially and environmentally responsible. The dual mission contrasts with other big science initiatives that focus principally or exclusively on technology development and application, such as the aforementioned Human Genome Project and, more recently, the National Institutes of Health (NIH) National Center for Advancing Translational Sciences (NCATS) and the multiagency Toxicity Testing in the 21st Century (Tox21) Initiative. Separation of applications research and implications research in those fields naturally allays concerns that the drive to commercialize emerging technologies could overshadow the fledgling understanding of possible risks. In nanotechnology, however, concerns regarding conflicts of interest between the dual objectives, the disparities in resource allocations, and the differential rate of research progress are important to a number of stakeholders.

Strong governance that separates the management of technology development from the management of EHS risk research is a potential solution. The risks associated with early-stage technology are intrinsically riddled with uncertainties; as this report alludes to in earlier chapters, the science needed to provide definitive answers is highly complex and integrative. Conclusions are not revealed in a single study but develop from a laborious and consistent set of work that may span years. When faced with the nuances of risk research, an organization that is in large measure evaluated by its success in technology development may not be perceived as able to set priorities effectively among either resources or topics for risk research.

If the potential research synergies and cross-fertilization between applications research and implications research are to be realized, concerns about the true equality of the dual objectives of "responsible development" must be addressed. Only then can all stakeholders trust that there is an equitable allocation of resources and an appropriate focus on the most risk-relevant questions.

One symptom of weak governance is the challenge of maintaining regular communication and coordination at all levels—between researchers in the United States, foreign researchers, and relevant stakeholders. In the United States, many research activities on ENMs have been under way for some time and are supported through coordinated efforts that include conferences and workshops. But the level of information-sharing and communication among the participants and with other stakeholders remains primarily informal and in the committee's judgment is insufficient. That is also true globally; effective alignment in nanotechnology EHS research strategies could provide enormous leverage to many countries that have active nanotechnology-research portfolios. It is important to recognize that constructive collaborative initiatives between the United States and the European Union are already under way (Finnish Institute of Occupational Health 2012).

With or without infusion of additional funds, the value of communication among investigators who are generating new nanomaterials and those who are studying EHS issues will need to be substantially improved. Improvements in collaboration and coordination among federal and nonfederal researchers would enhance the likelihood that research produces information that supports effective public-policy and private-sector decisions and ultimately protects the environment and human health. An integrated and well-coordinated program on both national and global scales would help to ensure that research findings provide the evidence needed to inform decisions so as to effectively manage and, ideally, prevent EHS risks. The continued challenges of communication and coordination, in spite of many good-faith efforts, are notable. There have been many efforts in the United States and abroad to identify and address research needs related to the safe use of nanotechnology but little continuity and follow-through to ensure that the needs are being addressed.

The committee summarizes below several core aspects of effective governance that reinforce recommendations that it offered in its first report (NRC 2012). The suggestions help to address the challenges of coordination among researchers, communication with external stakeholders, and perceptions of conflict of interest.

Empowered leadership. If all agencies are responsible, to some degree, for nanotechnology EHS research, no agency can be held clearly accountable for its management and progress. Our nation needs empowered leadership for nanotechnology risk research directed through a governance structure that clearly defines the metrics used to gauge progress and the roles and means of engagement of researchers and stakeholders. Without such leadership, efforts are likely to result in wasteful and duplicative efforts, fractured results, and knowledge gaps that could seriously dilute the science that underpins policy and regulatory decisions. Moreover, the gap in empowered leadership of nanotechnology EHS research at the federal level has made coordination and communication challenging and left the enterprise open to perceptions of conflicts between technology development and risk research.

Such leadership requires a stronger central convening authority than the NNI can now provide—one that has sufficient management and budgetary authority to direct implementation of a research strategy throughout all the NNI agencies and to ensure its integration with EHS research undertaken in the private sector, the academic community, and international organizations (NRC 2012, pp. 16-17). The committee recognizes that attaining that objective fully may require changes in the statute that established the NNI; as noted in our first report, such legislation was introduced but not adopted in the 111th Congress (NRC 2012, p. 166). Movement in the desired direction could be achieved through the designation of one of the NNI agencies whose mission includes EHS as the lead agency for directing EHS research throughout the federal government. Alternatively, it may be possible to establish a new entity to serve this function in analogy to the NIH NCATS.

Metrics of research progress. Delineation and tracking of clearly identified metrics of research progress are well suited to the capabilities of a central organization devoted to oversight of nanotechnology EHS research. Establishment of defined metrics that measure progress toward goals of a research strategy has been recommended by this committee (NRC 2012) and in other reviews of the NNI to increase the accountability of agencies and researchers. The specific needs include development and implementation of performance metrics that can be used to track research progress against core objectives, establishment of a rigorous means of assessing whether funded programs are conducting risk research, and periodic estimation of the levels and identification of the sources of funding needed to meet the specific goals and priorities defined by the agencies and the broader community.

As part of this activity, it is vital to strive for greater transparency in communicating the distribution of research in one's portfolio. Agencies need clearer guidance in differentiating between research directly relevant to EHS risk and applications-oriented research that has more indirect EHS implications. If research that centers on risk questions is clearly differentiated from research that develops applications with more distant EHS relevance, information on the relative amounts of funding allocated to the two will be viewed as more credible by many stakeholders.

Sustained coordination and communication with all relevant stakeholders. In spite of good-faith efforts, the committee finds that more structured, reliable, and continuing forums are needed both for communication among researchers (in the United States and globally) and for stakeholder engagement. For example, as uses of ENMs extend globally, research on the potential EHS consequences of ENMs should be considered globally. The committee's workshop that informed the present report provided a perspective on an extensive slate of research under way in Europe and elsewhere. The government should invest in such a way as to ensure that the research enterprise outlined in Figure 4-1 fully engages the global research community. Such engagement will widen the array of materials covered, provide analyses that address diverse and heterogeneous exposures and outcomes, and facilitate development of validated models.

Another important audience that needs to be engaged is stakeholders who are not part of the nanotechnology EHS research community. With that in mind, the committee has identified a number of attributes of effective stakeholder engagement that are largely missing from the NNI's efforts. It is especially important to provide a process to continuously engage stakeholders and to receive their input on research progress and priorities. That could be accomplished through, for example, the establishment of standing advisory bodies that meet regularly to review strategy development, implementation, and priorities. Such stakeholder groups may be best formed around application-specific sectors of nanotechnology and nanomaterials and encompass each of the links in the value chain (for example, workers, consumers, environmental advocates, and producers of raw materials, intermediates, and final products). As an initial step, the committee recommends that the National Nanotechnology Coordination Office (NNCO) establish its own stakeholder advisory council to develop best practices for this vital function and commit to funding regular workshops to bring together US and foreign researchers who are working on nanotechnology EHS research and other stakeholders.

Public–private partnerships. Engagement with stakeholders is important for shaping research on nanotechnology-related risk, but it does not fully leverage the opportunity to expand and enrich risk research through focused partnerships with them. To implement the ambitious strategies outlined by the NNI effectively, this committee and others will require substantial leveraging of federal funds, and the committee believes that public–private partnerships need to be more fully developed. Not only do such structures create the potential for greater resources, but direct stakeholder participation in partnerships that have defined research or communication goals is optimal for engagement.

The committee has identified five elements that are critical for effective public–private partnerships: a strong independent and accountable governance structure that provides transparency in selecting projects, conducting research, ensuring quality, and disseminating results; commitments of adequate and shared funding; open processes to develop priorities and specific goals; transparent sharing and peer review of research, including a commitment to release all research results and underlying data (NRC 2012, p. 173); and confidentiality agreements that balance the proprietary needs of industry participants with the public need to share information and make decision-making processes transparent.

Minimizing the potential for conflicts between applications research and implications research. The committee maintains that the NNI would benefit from a clearer separation of authority and accountability for its EHS research enterprise and its mandate to promote nanotechnology development and commercialization. The committee also acknowledges that, in the absence of a change in its statutory mandate, establishment of wholly separate management and budgetary structures and authorities for the NNI's dual functions may not be realistic. Nonetheless, steps can be taken at both the agency level and across the initiative as a whole to address this concern.

Agencies should create and adhere to strong scientific-integrity policies that govern both intramural and extramural research and should consider creating an ombudsman position to receive, investigate, and resolve complaints or concerns about bias and conflicts of interest related to nanotechnology research.

The NNCO should also develop and disseminate best practices for identifying, managing, and preventing conflicts of interest and bias in the planning, conduct, and reporting of research. Different offices and senior staff members that have parallel and comparable degrees of authority should be independently responsible for program management of the two lines of research within an agency. Moreover, agency scientists trained in the health or environmental sciences should be engaged in management of EHS risk-related research where possible.

SUSTAINING AND NURTURING RESEARCH EXCELLENCE

Whatever organization oversees the nanotechnology EHS research strategy, among its most important functions will be to secure and maintain adequate funding for the program. The research strategies outlined by the NNI and by this committee cannot be accomplished without a sustained commitment over at least the next decade. Such an investment will yield a more acceptable and ultimately more successful nanotechnology economy. It is only through a clear understanding of the scientific data and uncertainties that possible EHS risks posed by ENMs can be reduced. Such information accelerates nanotechnology development, lowers barriers to the introduction of new nanotechnology-containing products in the marketplace, and ensures public trust in the regulatory processes that protect the health of workers, the public, and the environment.

Multiple sources of funding are needed to support the research strategy, but a sustained high level of management and funding through a single agency is needed if indeed the critical research on EHS is to be accomplished. A successful knowledge commons requires strong leadership. Such commitments of funding will not be possible in the absence of a lead agency or organization that sees the issues as an essential part of its mission. Without such a lead organization to sustain support for the EHS agenda in the competition for government resources, the EHS nanotechnology research enterprise will falter, and we will not be able to achieve the ideal of responsible nanotechnology development.

Funding is only part of the challenge, however; it is vital that the best researchers in this country and beyond remain interested in and willing to tackle this problem. Various cultures in government, academe, and industry both support and sustain individual scientists and investigative teams. "Cultural and institutional obstacles often discourage attempts to perform research across disciplines, agencies, and institutions (including public and private organizations). Such obstacles can reflect historical tendencies to conduct research within particular disciplinary or organizational boundaries—for example, toxicology vs epidemiology and government vs industry" (NRC 2001, p. 141). Moreover, a scientist's career advancement requires attention to institutional, rather than national, agendas. A role as coauthor of a multidisciplinary manuscript may do little to advance an academic career if recognition is attached only to first or senior authorship. Similarly, scientific journals typically focus on particular fields and are reluctant to publish outside of their own scopes. Meetings of professional societies often run parallel sessions with researchers partitioned into focused sessions on physical science or biologic science, and this limits opportunities for cross-fertilization. All those factors taken together make it difficult to assemble the best teams to tackle the research outlined in Chapter 4.

In recognizing such disincentives as they apply to multidisciplinary research on EHS aspects of ENMs, the committee recommends that incentives be established to foster joint planning and information exchange. Examples of such incentives are enhanced support to give higher priority to multidisciplinary, integrated EHS aspects of ENMs; frequent multisponsor, multidisciplinary meetings to build a community of investigators addressing EHS aspects of ENMs; and a cross-agency budget for key multidisciplinary research initiatives. Such efforts might go a long way toward eliminating or at least decreasing the barriers that limit the broad perspective required in tackling the complex subject of EHS aspects of ENMs.

ADAPTIVE DECISION-MAKING AND KNOWLEDGE-SHARING

All stakeholders in nanotechnology EHS research, whether they are citizens or academic researchers, should have access to the growing body of knowledge surrounding nanotechnology-related EHS concerns. Such a resource would help to improve public understanding, inform policy-makers, offer data for future researchers, and shape the future focus of the research. As envisioned in Chapter 4, the diverse audiences would be served by the same resource—termed a knowledge commons—because it would provide information relevant to nanotechnology EHS research at multiple levels of detail. The resource would also provide an archival function: all data collected during the course of nanotechnology EHS research would be available to future generations of researchers.

For researchers, the most important aspect of the knowledge commons is access to existing data. The knowledge commons would provide storage for raw data or links to data derived from the processed data and would offer some curation, annotation, and linkages of datasets. Those features would make it possible to establish the provenance, reproducibility, and uncertainty of future data and in effect "bank" them for consideration by future researchers. The knowledge commons would provide a means of augmenting the current print literature digitally to access and compare raw data; evaluate their quality, uncertainty, and reproducibility; and augment collaboration to evaluate risk associated with both applications and implications of nanotechnology (Priem 2013). As presented in Chapter 4, research on nanotechnology-related risk is a highly multidisciplinary, systems-level scientific challenge; shared databases and knowledge commons are vital for rapid progress in that they permit the integration of information among material types, species, and exposure routes.

For interested stakeholders (such as regulators, scientists, workers, and consumers) who are not actively engaged in the research, the knowledge commons could serve as an excellent resource for meta-analysis of multiple publications, continuing research projects, and datasets. Summaries of research projects that lay out the key participants, goals, methods, models, underlying hypotheses, resource levels, schedules, and expected deliverables, and resulting publications or other avenues to access findings could be vital for adapting the priorities of nanotechnology EHS research in the United States. The availability of such information on line and regularly updated would serve to stimulate interactions, identify gaps, and avoid unnecessary duplication by researchers. It would also facilitate oversight of the nanomaterial research program and provide greater accountability for research progress. It may be possible to engage researchers to offer snapshots or meta-analyses of the state of knowledge in their own fields, and this information could feed into an adaptive decision-making process that constantly evaluates the evolving consensus developing in the research community on such key issues as those presented in Chapter 4.

Finally, the knowledge commons would provide context for addressing and satisfying the widely recognized need for improved terminology for ENM structures, experiments, characteristics, models, effects, and uses. It is vital that the terminology used in one study be compatible with that used in other studies. An ideal solution envisions a common taxonomy for all nanomaterials, methods, and risk-related data; however, attempts at even the simplest nomenclature have been under way for years and have yet to yield universally accepted definitions of even the most basic ENMs.

A more pragmatic approach would be to develop ontologies and thesauruses that in effect map a given set of defined terms onto other commonly used sets to permit data to be fully shared even if researchers in different disciplines adopt different conventions for nomenclature formatting and reporting. Bioinformatics provides relevant examples of what can be accomplished with these techniques; for example, the National Cancer Institute's Metathesaurus provides synonyms that link cancer research and trial resources (NCI 2013) and linkages to hundreds of resources accessible through the National Library of Medicine (NLM 2013). There is far less controversy in defining ontologies for particular domains of knowledge and practice, but ontologies require the deep engagement of the research community in mapping terms among disciplines, conventions, and business practices. Without such tools, progress toward the ideal laid out in Chapter 4 and the NNI's own research strategy will be severely compromised.

Ultimately, the goal would be to encourage all researchers to label and organize their materials by using one of several accepted and defined ontologies. There will need to be a working convention that describes target materials of interest and presents several options for their nomenclature. The terminology challenge extends to the description of the key characteristics and properties of ENMs at different levels of granularity—from atomistic and molecular through single particles, aggregates, structures, and systems for use in experiments, models, manufacture, and application. ENMs' properties determine their novel or enhanced physical, chemical, and biologic behavior, and future definitions can incorporate readily measurable properties, such as particle diameter and size distribution. Decision-makers charged in the near term with inventorying or registering ENMs have sometimes adopted definitions out of necessity, and these frameworks could be the basis of ontologies. If those approaches are coupled with the ability to adapt rapidly to new findings or growing consensus in the research community, they are likely to become widely adopted.

Ontologies are tools for researchers and should not be used to generalize ENM properties or risks. As has been shown in multiple studies, the starting features of an ENM are only a few of the many attributes that define their actions in biologic or environmental systems. As scientific understanding grows, the best terms for describing ENM properties will become clearer to the community. Ontologies provide an excellent approach for capturing that evolution in that they will allow publications from the 1990s to be related to more recent literature. However, achieving such results will require continuing investment in not only the informatics infrastructure but the personnel required to maintain the enterprise: the data scientists, curators, and informaticists necessary to define terms authoritatively, evaluate the quality and reproducibility of experimental data and models, conduct validations, and aid users. Support of these activities by research scientists will be necessary, particularly in providing expert opinion and analyses. Equally important is the recognition that informatics specialists provide crucial capabilities for planning, developing, and using the infrastructure discussed here (Monastersky 2013).

CONCLUSION

Characterization of the risks posed by ENMs throughout their life cycle is a scientific challenge that requires integrated, quantitative, and systems-level approaches. It is also an institutional challenge that stretches the conventional roles of agencies and researchers alike. Strong governance will be vital for ensuring effective, timely, and actionable research results. Ideally, empowered leadership at the federal level with oversight by a single agency would solve many of the organizational barriers perceived by the committee. Centralized attention to the arguments for sustained funding for this research and for the infrastructure needed to support data-sharing would be wise investments. The ideal of responsible development of nanotechnology is both daunting, but there is no doubt that it is attainable if we plan well for the substance of the research and for the management infrastructure needed to shape and disseminate its findings.

REFERENCES

Finnish Institute of Occupational Health. 2012. EU-U.S. nanoEHS Community of Research (CORs) Flyer [online]. Available: http://www.nanosustain.eu/events/COR%20flyer.pdf [accessed Feb. 1, 2013].

Hutchinson, J.E. 2008. Greener nanoscience: A proactive approach to advancing applications and reducing implication of nanotechnology. ACS Nano 2(3):395-402.

Monastersky, R. 2013. The library reboot. Nature. 495(7442):430-432.

NCI (National Cancer Institute). 2013. NCI Metathesaurus (NClm). Biomedical Terminology Database. Version 2.2 [online]. Available: http://ncim.nci.nih.gov/ncimbrowser/ [accessed Mar. 29, 2013].

NIOSH (National Institute for Occupational Safety and Health). 2012. Prevention through Design. Workplace Safety and Health Topics [online]. Available: http://www.cdc.gov/niosh/topics/ptd/ [accessed Mar. 20, 2013].

NLM (National Library of Medicine). 2013. Databases, Resources, & APIs [online]. Available: http://wwwcf2.nlm.nih.gov/nlm_eresources/eresources/search_database.cfm [accessed Mar. 29, 2013].

NRC (National Research Council). 2001. Research Priorities for Airborne Particulate Matter: III. Early Research Progress. Washington, DC: National Academy Press.

NRC (National Research Council). 2012. A Research Strategy for Environmental, Health, and Safety Aspects of Engineered Nanomaterials. Washington, DC: National Academies Press.

Priem, J. 2013. Beyond the paper. Nature. 495(7442):437-440.

Appendix A

Biographic Information on the Committee to Develop A Research Strategy For Environmental, Health, and Safety Aspects of Engineered Nanomaterials

JONATHAN M. SAMET (*Chair*) is a pulmonary physician and epidemiologist. He is a professor and Flora L. Thornton Chair of the Department of Preventive Medicine of the Keck School of Medicine of the University of Southern California (USC) and director of the USC Institute for Global Health. Dr. Samet's research has focused on the health risks posed by inhaled pollutants. He has served on numerous committees concerned with public health: the U.S. Environmental Protection Agency Science Advisory Board; committees of the National Research Council, including chairing the Committee on Biological Effects of Ionizing Radiation VI, the Committee on Research Priorities for Airborne Particulate Matter, and the Board on Environmental Studies and Toxicology; and committees of the Institute of Medicine (IOM). He is a member of IOM. Dr. Samet received his MD from the University of Rochester School of Medicine and Dentistry.

JURRON BRADLEY joined BASF as a clean energy market manager in June 2011. In this role, he is responsible for creating BASF's first market facing-unit for the clean energy industry. Before joining BASF, Jurron led the consulting team at Lux Research, which provides clients with strategic advice on technology, including nanotechnology, and market trends and themes. Before joining Lux Research, Dr. Bradley worked at Praxair, Inc., where he designed air separation and argon recycling plants and managed a thermodynamics laboratory. He also led research efforts to reduce mercury emissions from coal-fired boilers and worked on the development of technology to reduce emissions of nitrogen oxides from coal-fired boilers. Dr. Bradley later joined Praxair's technology planning and strategy group in which he played a key role in developing strategic approaches for the entire research and development organization. Dr. Bradley received a PhD in chemical engineering from the Georgia Institute of Technology.

SETH COE-SULLIVAN is a cofounder and chief technology officer of QD Vision. His work spans quantum dot materials; new fabrication techniques, including thin-film deposition equipment design; and device architectures for efficient QD-LED light emission. Dr. Coe-Sullivan has more than 20 papers and patents pending in the fields of organic light-emitting devices, quantum dot LEDs, and nanotechnology fabrication. He was awarded *Technology Review* magazine's TR35 Award in 2006 as one of the top 35 innovators under the age of 35 years. In 2007, *BusinessWeek* named him one of the top young entrepreneurs under the age of 30 years, and in 2009, he was a finalist for the Mass Technology Leadership Council's CTO of the year. Dr. Coe-Sullivan serves on Brown University's Engineering Advisory Council. He received his PhD in electrical engineering from the Massachusetts Institute of Technology; his thesis work on incorporating quantum dots into hybrid organic-inorganic LED structures led to the formation of QD Vision.

VICKI L. COLVIN is vice provost for research, professor of chemistry, and director of the Center for Biological and Environmental Nanotechnology (CBEN) at Rice University. Among CBEN's primary interests is the application of nanotechnology to the environment. She has received numerous accolades for her teaching abilities, including Phi Beta Kappa's Teaching Prize for 1998-1999 and the Camille Dreyfus Teacher Scholar Award in 2002. In 2002, she was also named one of *Discover* magazine's Top 20 Scientists to Watch and received an Alfred P. Sloan Fellowship. In 2007, she was named a fellow of the American Association for the Advancement of Science (AAAS). Dr. Colvin is a frequent contributor to *Advanced Materials*, *Physical Review Letters*, and other peer-reviewed journals and holds patents to seven inventions. Dr. Colvin served on the NRC Committee for Review of the Federal Strategy to Address Environmental, Health, and Safety Research Needs for Engineered Nanoscale Materials. She received her PhD in chemistry from the University of California, Berkeley, where she was awarded the American Chemical Society's Victor K. LaMer Award for her work in colloid and surface chemistry.

EDWARD D. CRANDALL is the Hastings Professor and Kenneth T. Norris, Jr. Chair of Medicine and chair of the Division of Pulmonary and Critical Care Medicine of the Keck School of Medicine of the University of Southern California. Dr. Crandall's clinical interests include critical-care medicine and pulmonary disease. He has written numerous peer-reviewed articles on cardiopulmonary biology. His specific research interests are in the regulation of the differentiation and transport properties of alveolar epithelial cells. He is actively involved in research on the interactions of nanomaterials with alveolar epithelium. Dr. Crandall received his PhD from Northwestern University and his MD from the University of Pennsylvania.

RICHARD A. DENISON is a senior scientist at the Environmental Defense Fund. Dr. Denison has 28 years of experience in the environmental arena, specializing in chemical policy and hazards, exposure, and risk assessment and management of industrial chemicals and nanomaterials. He has testified before Congress numerous times on the need for fundamental reform of US policy toward industrial chemicals and on nanomaterial safety research needs. Dr. Denison is a member of the NRC Standing Committee on Emerging Science for Environmental Health Decisions and until recently served on the NRC Board on Environmental Studies and Toxicology. He serves on the Green Ribbon Science Panel for California's Green Chemistry Initiative, and was a member of the National Pollution Prevention and Toxics Advisory Committee, which advised the Environmental Protection Agency's Office of Pollution Prevention and Toxics. He was a member of EDF's team that worked jointly with the DuPont Corporation to develop a framework governing responsible development, production, use, and disposal of nanoscale materials. Previously, Dr. Denison was an analyst and assistant project director in the Oceans and Environment Program of the Office of Technology Assessment of the U.S. Congress. Dr. Denison received his PhD in molecular biophysics and biochemistry from Yale University.

WILLIAM H. FARLAND is the senior vice president for research of Colorado State University and a professor in its Department of Environmental and Radiological Health Sciences in the School of Veterinary Medicine and Biomedical Sciences. In 2006, Dr. Farland was appointed deputy assistant administrator for science in the Environmental Protection Agency (EPA) Office of Research and Development (ORD). He had served as the acting deputy assistant administrator since 2001. In 2003, Dr. Farland has also been chief scientist in the Office of the Agency Science Adviser. He served as EPA's acting science adviser throughout 2005. Formerly, he was the director of ORD National Center for Environmental Assessment. Dr. Farland served on a number of executive-level committees and advisory boards in the federal government. In 2005-2006, he chaired the Executive Committee of the National Toxicology Program. He was also a member of the Scientific Advisory Council of the Risk Sciences and Public Policy Institute of the Johns Hopkins University School of Hygiene and Public Health, a public member of the American Chemistry Council's Strategic Science Team for its Long-Range Research Initiative, and a member of the Programme Advisory Committee for the World Health Organization's International Programme on Chemical Safety. Dr. Farland recently served as chair of an external advisory group for the National Institute of Environmental Health Sciences regarding the future of the Superfund Basic Research Program. He is the chair of a standing Committee on Emerging Science for Environmental Health Decisions of the National Research Council. In 2002, Dr. Farland was recognized by the Society for Risk Analysis with the Outstanding Risk Practitioner Award, and in 2005, he was named a fellow of the society. In 2006, he received a Presidential Rank Award for his service as a federal senior executive. In 2007, he was elected a fellow of the Academy of Toxicological Sciences. Dr. Farland received his PhD from the University of California, Los Angeles in cell biology and biochemistry.

MARTIN FRITTS is an emeritus researcher at SAIC-Frederick, Frederick National Laboratory for Cancer Research (FNLCR), and a research associate in the Materials Measurement Laboratory at the National Institute of Standards and Technology (NIST). Dr. Fritts supported SAIC-Frederick in implementing the National Cancer Institute's Cancer Nanotechnology Plan and the establishment of the Nanotechnology Characterization Laboratory at the FNLCR, and he works with NIST in their programs in nanotechnology, informatics, and the Materials Genome Initiative. His primary interests are in the development of advanced imaging and measurement instrumentation, modeling, and simulation to elucidate structure-activity relationships of nanomaterials in biologic environments, and informatics systems to aid in improving data quality and advance knowledge-sharing. Dr. Fritts also serves as the cochair of the American Society for Testing and Materials' E56.02 Subcommittee on Nanotechnology Characterization, and is a member of American National Standards Institute's US Technical Advisory Group for ISO/TC 229, Nanotechnologies. Before joining SAIC-Frederick, he developed and prototyped nanotechnology applications for industry and government through SAIC's Nanotechnology Initiatives Division. His previous experience includes work in computational physics with the Naval Research Laboratory and with SAIC on computational fluid dynamics, simulation-based design, ship design, and nuclear fusion. His work has emphasized collaboration in science and its translation to applications in industry, academia, and government. Dr. Fritts earned a PhD in nuclear physics from Yale University.

PHILIP K. HOPKE is the Bayard D. Clarkson Distinguished Professor in the Department of Chemical and Biomolecular Engineering and the Department of Chemistry of Clarkson University. He is also director of the university's Center for the Environment and its Center for Air Resources Engineering and Sciences. His research interests are related primarily to particles in the air, including particle formation, sampling and analysis, composition, and origin. His current projects are related to receptor modeling, ambient monitoring, and nucleation. Dr. Hopke has been elected to membership in the International Statistics Institute and is a fellow of the American Association for the Advancement of Science. He is also a fellow of the American Association for Aerosol Research, in which he has served in various roles, including president, vice president, and member of the board of directors. Dr. Hopke is a member of the American Institute of Chemical Engineers, the International Society of Exposure Science, and the International Society of Indoor Air Quality and Climate, and others. He has served as a member of the U.S. Environmental Protection Agency Advisory Council on Clean Air Act Compliance Analysis and as a member of several National Research Council committees, most recently the Committee on Energy Futures and Air Pollution in Urban China and the United States, the Committee on Research Priorities for Airborne Particulate Matter, and the Committee on Air Quality

Management in the United States. Dr. Hopke received his PhD in chemistry from Princeton University.

JAMES E. HUTCHISON is the Lokey-Harrington Professor of Chemistry at the University of Oregon. He is the founding director of the Oregon Nanoscience and Microtechnologies Institute for Safer Nanomaterials and Nanomanufacturing Initiative, a virtual center that unites 30 principal investigators in the Northwest around the goals of designing greener nanomaterials and nanomanufacturing. Dr. Hutchison's research focuses on molecular-level design and synthesis of functional surface coatings and nanomaterials for a wide array of applications, in which the design of new processes and materials draws heavily on the principles of green chemistry. Dr. Hutchison received several awards and honors, including the Alfred P. Sloan Research Fellowship and the National Science Foundation CAREER Award. He was a member of the National Research Council Committee on Grand Challenges for Sustainability in the Chemistry Industry. Dr. Hutchison received his PhD in organic chemistry from Stanford University.

REBECCA D. KLAPER is an associate professor in the School of Freshwater Sciences, University of Wisconsin-Milwaukee. The School of Freshwater Sciences (at the Great Lakes WATER Institute) is dedicated to providing basic and applied research to inform policy decisions involving freshwater resources. Dr. Klaper uses traditional toxicologic methods and genomic technologies to study the potential effects of emerging contaminants, such as nanoparticles and pharmaceuticals, on aquatic organisms. Dr. Klaper received an American Association for the Advancement of Science and Technology Policy Fellowship, in which she worked in the National Center for Environmental Assessment at the Environmental Protection Agency (EPA). She has served as an invited scientific expert to both the U.S. National Nanotechnology Initiative and the Organisation for Economic and Co-operative Development Panel on Nanotechnology, for which she has testified on the potential effects of nanoparticles on the environment and the utility of current testing strategies. She has served as a technical expert in reviewing the EPA white paper on the environmental effects of nanotechnologies and the EPA research strategy for nanotechnology. She also was involved in writing the EPA white paper on the use of genomic technologies in risk assessment. Dr. Klaper received her PhD in ecology from the Institute of Ecology of the University of Georgia.

GREGORY V. LOWRY is a professor in the Department of Civil and Environmental Engineering of Carnegie Mellon University and deputy director of the National Science Foundation Center for Environmental Implications of Nanotechnology. He researches sustainable development of nanomaterials and nanotechnologies, including the fate, mobility, and toxicity of nanomaterials in the environment, remediation and treatment technologies that use nanomaterials, and nanoparticle-contaminant and biota interactions. He also works on sustainable energy via carbon capture and storage. His current projects include elucidating the role of adsorbed macromolecules on nanoparticle transport and fate in the environment, in situ sediment management with innovative sediment caps, dense nonaqueous-phase liquid source zone remediation through delivery of reactive nanoparticles to the nonaqueous-phase-water interface, and carbon dioxide capture, sequestration, and monitoring. Dr. Lowry served as an external advisory board member for the Center for Biological and Environmental Nanotechnology. He was a review panelist for the Environmental Protection Agency draft nanomaterial research strategy. He is a member of the American Chemical Society, the American Society of Civil Engineers, and the Association of Environmental Engineering and Science Professors. He received his PhD in civil-environmental engineering from Stanford University.

ANDREW D. MAYNARD is the director of the Risk Science Center of the University of Michigan School of Public Health. He previously served as the chief science adviser in the Woodrow Wilson International Center for Scholars for the Project on Emerging Nanotechnologies. Dr. Maynard's research interests revolve around aerosol characterization, the implications of nanotechnology for human health and the environment, and managing the challenges and opportunities of emerging technologies. Dr. Maynard's expertise covers many facets of risk science, emerging technologies, science policy, and communication. Previously, he worked for the National Institute for Occupational Safety and Health and represented the agency on the Nanomaterial Science, Engineering and Technology (NSET) subcommittee of the National Science and Technology Council and cochaired the Nanotechnology Health and Environment Implications working group of NSET. He serves on the World Economic Forum Global Agenda Council on Emerging Technologies and is a member of the Executive Committee of the International Council on Nanotechnology. He previously chaired the International Standards Organization Working Group on size-selective sampling in the workplace. Dr. Maynard served as a member of the NRC Committee for Review of the Federal Strategy to Address Environmental, Health, and Safety Research Needs for Engineered Nanoscale Materials. He earned his PhD in aerosol physics from the Cavendish Laboratory of the University of Cambridge, UK.

GÜNTER OBERDÖRSTER is a professor in the Department of Environmental Medicine of the University of Rochester, director of the University of Rochester Ultrafine Particle Center, principal investigator of a Multidisciplinary Research Initiative in Nanotoxicology, and head of the Pulmonary Core of the National Institute of Environmental Health Sciences Center Grant. His research includes the effects and underlying mechanisms of lung injury induced by inhaled nonfibrous and fibrous particles, including extrapolation modeling and risk assessment. His studies with ultrafine particles influenced the field of inhalation toxicology, raising awareness of the unique biokinetics and toxic potential of nano-sized particles. He has served on many national and international committees and is the recipient of several scientific awards. Dr. Oberdörster has served on several National Research Council committees, including the Committee on Research Priorities for Airborne Particulate Matter and the Committee on the Review of the Federal Strategy to Address Environmental, Health, and Safety Research Needs for Engineered Nanoscale Materials. He is on the editorial boards of the *Journal of Aerosol Medicine, Particle and Fibre Toxicology, Nanotoxicology,* and the *International Journal of Hygiene and Environmental Health* and is associate editor of *Inhalation Toxicology* and *Environmental Health Perspectives*. He earned his DVM and PhD (in pharmacology) from the University of Giessen, Germany.

KATHLEEN M. REST is the executive director of the Union of Concerned Scientists (UCS), a science-based nonprofit. She manages the organization's day-to-day affairs, supervising programs on issues ranging from climate change and clean energy to global security. Dr. Rest came to UCS from the National Institute for Occupational Safety and Health (NIOSH) in the Centers for Disease Control and Prevention, where she was the deputy director for programs. Throughout her tenure at NIOSH, she held several leadership positions, including serving as the institute's acting director during the period of September 11, 2001, and the anthrax events that followed. Before her federal service, Dr. Rest served on the faculty of several medical schools—most recently as an associate professor in the Department of Family and Community Medicine of the University of Massachusetts Medical Center and an adjunct associate professor in the University of Massachusetts School of Public Health—where she taught occupational, environmental, and public health. She has extensive experience as a researcher and adviser on occupational and environmental health issues in various countries, such as the Netherlands, Slovakia, Poland, Romania, Canada, and Greece. Dr. Rest was a founding member of the Association of Occupational and Environmental Clinics, a national nonprofit organization committed to improving the practice of occupational and environmental health through information-sharing and collaborative research. She also served as the chairperson of the National Advisory Committee on Occupational Safety and Health. Dr. Rest earned her PhD in health policy from Boston University.

MARK J. UTELL is a professor of medicine and environmental medicine, a director of occupational and environmental medicine, and former director of pulmonary and critical-care medicine in the University of Rochester Medical Center. He serves as associate chairman of the Department of Environmental Medicine. His research interests have centered on the effects of environmental toxicants on the human respiratory tract. Dr. Utell has published extensively on the health effects of inhaled gases, particles, and fibers in the workplace and other indoor and outdoor environments. He is the co-principal investigator of an Environmental Protection Agency (EPA) Particulate Matter Center and chair of the Health Effects Institute's Research Committee. He has served as chair of EPA's Environmental Health Committee and on the Executive Committee of the

EPA Science Advisory Board. He is a former recipient of the National Institute of Environmental Health Sciences Academic Award in Environmental and Occupational Medicine. Dr. Utell is currently a member of the National Research Council's Board on Environmental Studies and Toxicology. He previously served on the National Research Council Committee on Research Priorities for Airborne Particulate Matter, the Institute of Medicine (IOM) Committee to Review the Health Consequences of Service during the Persian Gulf War, and the IOM Committee on Biodefense Analysis and Countermeasures. He received his MD from Tufts University School of Medicine.

DAVID B. WARHEIT received his PhD in physiology from Wayne State University School of Medicine in Detroit. Later, he received a National Institutes of Health (NIH) postdoctoral fellowship, and 2 years later, a Parker Francis Pulmonary Fellowship, both of which he took to the National Institute of Environmental Health Sciences to study mechanisms of asbestos-related lung disease with Arnold Brody. In 1984, he moved to the DuPont Haskell Laboratory to develop a pulmonary-toxicology research laboratory. His major research interests are pulmonary toxicity mechanisms and corresponding risks related to inhaled particles, fibers, and nanomaterials. He is the author or coauthor of more than 100 publications and has been the recipient of the International Life Sciences Institute (ILSI) Kenneth Morgareidge Award (1993, Hannover, Germany) for contributions in toxicology by a young investigator and the Robert A. Scala Award and Lectureship in Toxicology (2000). He has also attained diplomate status of the Academy of Toxicological Sciences (2000) and the American Board of Toxicology (1988). He has served on NIH review committees (NIH Small Business Innovation Research and NIH Bioengineering) and has participated in working groups of the International Agency for Research on Cancer, the European Centre for Ecotoxicology and Toxicology of Chemicals, Organisation for Economic Co-operation and Development, the ILSI Risk Science Institute, the ILSI Health and Environmental Sciences Institute, and the National Research Council. He has served on several journal editorial boards, including *Inhalation Toxicology and Toxicological Sciences* (as the current associate editor), *Particle and Fibre Toxicology*, *Toxicology Letters,* and *Nano Letters*. He is the chairman of the European Centre for Ecotoxicology and Toxicology of Chemicals Task Force on Health and Environmental Safety of Nanomaterials, serves on the National Institute for Occupational Safety and Health Board of Scientific Counselors, and is interim vice-president of the Nanotoxicology Specialty Section.

MARK R. WIESNER serves as director of the Center for the Environmental Implications of Nanotechnology, headquartered at Duke University, where he holds the James L. Meriam Chair in Civil and Environmental Engineering with appointments in the Pratt School of Engineering and the Nicholas School of Environment. Dr. Wiesner's research has focused on the applications of emerging nanomaterials to membrane science and water treatment and an examination of the fate, transport, and effects of nanomaterials in the environment. He was coeditor and author of *Environmental Nanotechnologies* and serves as associate editor of the journals *Nanotoxicology* and *Environmental Engineering Science*. Before joining the Duke University faculty in 2006, Dr.Wiesner was a member of the Rice University faculty for 18 years, where he held appointments in the Department of Civil and Environmental Engineering and the Department of Chemical Engineering and served as associate dean of engineering and director of the Environmental and Energy Systems Institute. Before working in academe, Dr. Wiesner was a research engineer with the French company Lyonnaise des Eaux, in Le Pecq, France, and a principal engineer with the environmental engineering consulting firm of Malcolm Pirnie, Inc., White Plains, NY. He received the1995 Rudolf Hering Medal from the American Society of Civil Engineers, of which he is a fellow, and the 2004 Frontiers in Research Award from the Association of Environmental Engineering and Science Professors, on whose board he serves. In 2004, Dr. Wiesner was also named a de Fermat Laureate and was awarded an International Chair of Excellence in the Chemical Engineering Laboratory of the French Polytechnic Institute and National Institute for Applied Sciences in Toulouse, France. He received his PhD in environmental engineering from the Johns Hopkins University.

Appendix B

Statement of Task

The National Research Council will develop and will monitor the implementation of an integrated research strategy to address the environmental, health, and safety aspects of engineered nanomaterials. This study will create a conceptual framework for environmental, health, and safety-related research; develop a research plan with short- and long-term research priorities; estimate resources necessary to implement this research plan; and subsequently evaluate research progress over a three year period. The committee will take into consideration current and emerging uses of engineered nanomaterials and the scientific uncertainties related to physical and chemical properties, potential exposures, toxicity, toxicokinetics, and environmental fate of these materials. In its evaluation the committee will also consider existing research roadmaps and progress made in their implementation.

Two reports will be prepared over a 4-year period. The first report, which will be released within 18 months of study inception, will present a conceptual framework and priorities for the research program, identify the most important short-term and longer-term research priorities, develop a strategy for monitoring and evaluating research progress, and estimate the resources needed to implement this strategy. A second and final report at the end of the study will evaluate research progress and update the research priorities and resource estimates based on results of studies and emerging trends in the nanotechnology industry. The committee will not estimate actual risks or benefits associated with environmental, health, and safety aspects of nanomaterials.

The first report will consider:

- What properties of engineered nanomaterials need to be considered to assess their potential exposures, toxicity, toxicokinetics, and environmental fate? What standardization of testing materials is needed?

- What methods and technologies are needed for detecting, measuring, analyzing, and monitoring engineered nanomaterials? What gaps in analytical capability need to be addressed?
- What exposure, toxicology, toxicokinetic, human health and environmental fate studies are needed for assessing the risks of engineered nanomaterials?
- What testing methods should be developed for assessing the potential toxicity, toxicokinetics, and environmental fate of engineered nanomaterials?
- What models should be developed for predicting the impacts of engineered nanomaterials on human health and the environment?
- What are the research priorities for understanding lifecycle risks to humans and the environment from applications of nanotechnology?
- What criteria should be used to evaluate research progress?

The second report will address the following issues:

- What research progress has been made in understanding the health, environmental, and safety aspects of nanotechnology? How does the research progress affect relevance of the initial set of research priorities?
- How have market and regulatory conditions changed and how does this affect the research priorities?
- Are the criteria for evaluating the research progress on the health, environmental, and safety aspects of nanotechnology appropriate?
- Considering the criteria developed, to what extent have short-term and long-term research priorities been initiated and implemented?

Appendix C

Workshop Summary: Research Progress on Environmental, Health, and Safety Aspects of Nanotechnology

On November 7, 2012, the National Research Council Committee to Develop a Research Strategy for Environmental, Health, and Safety Aspects of Engineered Nanomaterials held a workshop to obtain input on research progress since release of the committee's first report, *A Research Strategy for Environmental, Health, and Safety Aspects of Engineered Nanomaterials* (NRC 2012) and to learn of other efforts that were under way to address scientific uncertainties and infrastructure needed for a robust approach to research on EHS issues related to ENMs. The workshop featured presentations by federal agency and foreign officials, academic researchers, and representatives of nongovernment organizations and industry on the scientific and regulatory framework for EHS research, on recent research progress, and on applications of the results of research to risk management. Panel discussions provided opportunities for expanded discussion of many of the issues raised during the presentations. The information gathered in the workshop informs the committee's present report.

Setting the Stage—Emerging Issues and Emerging Materials

In response to questions regarding the possible EHS risks posed by ENMs, the workshop documented increased efforts by government agencies—in particular the NNI, academic institutions, and industry—to investigate, translate, and communicate information on the environmental and health aspects of nanotechnology. This workshop was part of the committee's information-gathering effort to improve understanding of the evolving research landscape as it developed its report. In opening remarks to the workshop participants, Jonathan Samet, of the

University of Southern California, chair of the committee, reviewed the charge to the committee and key messages from the committee's first report, which was released in January 2012.

Maxine Savitz, a member of the President's Council of Advisors on Science and Technology, described the NNI's investment in nanotechnology and specifically in EHS research. She commented on recommendations in the *Report to the President and Congress on the Fourth Assessment of the National Nanotechnology Initiative* (PCAST 2012). Specifically, Dr. Savitz highlighted needs for a higher-level authority that is accountable for EHS research to ensure that better policy is made; for an increase in the EHS nanotechnology research budget to about $25 million in cross-cutting fields, including informatics and instrumentation development (a recommendation originally made in the present committee's first report); for an emphasis on partnerships and interagency collaborations; for greater attention to worker safety by industry; and for individual agencies to have implementation plans that result from the federal strategic plan.

Michael Holman, of Lux Research, described trends in nanotechnology commercialization. The nanotechnology industry is no longer focused on manufacture of novel nanomaterials but is interested in integrating the materials into intermediate products. For example, he commented that most of the industry's effort will focus not on novel material classes but on successful integration (and novel uses) of known nanomaterials—carbon nanotubes, metal nanoparticles, ceramic nanoparticles (silicon dioxide and aluminum and zinc oxides), quantum dots, nanostructured metals and ceramics, and nanoporous materials. Dr. Holman also described movement away from improvement of existing products to enabling new ones. The shift is evident in the solar and nanomedicine fields. In addition, small and large companies are shifting from emphasizing "nano per se" to emphasizing how nanotechnology innovations solve problems. For example, in 2002-2007, many large companies had central nanotechnology initiatives; now, nanotechnology activities are typically incorporated into the business (functional) teams. Startups are less likely to term themselves nanotech companies and more likely to define themselves by the applications of their products.

Jim Alwood, of the US Environmental Protection Agency (EPA) Office of Pollution Prevention and Toxics, reported that under the Toxics Substances Control Act more than 140 new chemical notices for ENMs have been received since 2005 (30 related to carbon nanotubes or fibers). However, Mr. Alwood, a regulator, commented that there is not much information on existing uses of ENMs and on what materials are being manufactured. He acknowledged that materials cannot be regulated case by case, but stated that categories of nanomaterials need to be developed, as happens in EPA's chemical program, and data on nanomaterials need to be integrated into risk assessments to identify those that are of concern for risk management. Mr. Alwood commented that the most important data needs are for characterization of ENMs and for understanding exposures.

Georgios Katalagarianakis, of the European Commission (EC), discussed initiatives in the European Union (EU), including the Communities of Research

(CoR) launched in a joint EU-US effort by the EC and the National Nanotechnology Coordination Office (NNCO), to address EHS questions about ENMs and to advance the field collaboratively.

Institutional Needs to Support the Research Enterprise

In its first report (NRC 2012), the committee identified institutional arrangements and mechanisms that need to be addressed better to support implementation of the research enterprise, including fostering interagency interaction, collaboration, and accountability; developing and implementing mechanisms for stakeholder engagement; advancing integration among sectors and institutions involved in EHS research, including public–private partnerships; and implementing structural changes aimed at conflicts of interest. Representatives of federal organizations—including Sally Tinkle, NNCO; Tina Bahadori, EPA; Christopher Weis, National Institute of Environmental Health Sciences (NIEHS); Charles Geraci, National Institute for Occupational Safety and Health (NIOSH); Mike Roco, National Science Foundation (NSF); Teresa Croce, US Food and Drug Administration (FDA); and Scott McNeil, National Cancer Institute (NCI)—addressed a number of those themes and provided examples of recent efforts.

Dr. Tinkle reviewed efforts to map the NNI's EHS research-strategy goals to its strategic plan; further mapping will occur in the NNI's supplement to the president's 2014 budget. The NNI is trying to establish a process for tracking research progress. Dr. Tinkle commented that the NNI is considering requesting an Office of Management and Budget data call-in every 3 years, as was conducted in 2006 and 2009, to obtain EHS nanotechnology project-by-project data from all the federal agencies' NNI projects. She stated that a much higher-level review would occur during the intervening years.

Dr. Weis described coordination efforts within NIEHS and with other federal agencies, including FDA, NIOSH, and EPA. He commented on the successful coordination involved in the development of the NIEHS strategic plan, which is now being implemented, and emphasized that quality assurance and careful characterization of ENMs are needed for communication and exchange of data and findings.

Dr. Geraci discussed how NIOSH's work is closely aligned with that of other agencies' goals and how NIOSH coordinates with the NNI and external partners in the private, academic, government, and international sectors. He described efforts aimed at stakeholder engagement, including direct engagement with the nanomaterial industry through the site-visit program for nanomaterial manufacture and use and through evaluation of materials and processes that are under development. Dr. Geraci also described efforts to communicate results from NIOSH public–private partnerships, including publication of research results from NIOSH and development of memoranda of understanding at key research and development centers; he stated that further development of public–private interactions is needed.

Dr. McNeil reported that NCI–Frederick (now called the Frederick National Laboratory for Cancer Research or the Frederick National Lab [Reynolds 2012]) recently became a national laboratory and is able to conduct research through public–private partnerships and with other agencies. It offers a niche where material scientists, toxicologists, and others can, for example, examine specific questions regarding interactions between nanomaterials and biologic systems. Dr. McNeil provided several examples of the laboratory's work with NIEHS and FDA on nanomaterials and an industry partnership to assess toxicity of nanocrystalline cellulose.

Perspectives of Researchers

Several researchers discussed directions and initiatives that they considered to have the highest priority for addressing uncertainties about EHS aspects of ENMs. Martin Philbert, of the University of Michigan School of Public Health, discussed the need to learn lessons from nanomedicine, emphasizing that drug development takes longer than it used to and that public–private partnerships are needed. He suggested the need to consider the "rule of six" for nanotechnology EHS research that was originally developed to move clinical drug development forward by identifying a simple set of physicochemical parameter ranges that the compounds needed to meet for design and selection (see Keller et al. 2006). He emphasized that there are few chronic safety studies on ENMs and that we need to move beyond classical toxicology to less expensive, higher-throughput analyses.

Robert Tanguay, of Oregon State University, noted that ENM behavior depends completely on a material's inherent properties and that the goal of EHS research is to develop methods for predicting behaviors from the inherent properties. He described progress toward filling research gaps: distribution of some reference materials and their use in cross-evaluation of models, wider acceptance of minimum characterization standards (although perhaps not yet sufficient), greater understanding of the dynamic behavior of ENMs, greater understanding of the need for precision engineering to support structure–response relationship studies, and application of Tox21[1] principles to in vitro and in vivo studies (for example, in zebrafish). However, the focus remains on simple materials with a heavy emphasis on silver ENMs and metal oxides. Apart from that progress, Dr. Tanguay commented that the key toxicologic question remains: What are the unique properties that influence toxicity? Dr. Tanguay described research that is needed to explore the unique properties of ENMs systematically and to understand how these properties influence molecular interactions and biocompatibility. The needs include further development of characterization

---

[1]Tox21 is a collaboration among EPA, NIEHS, the National Human Genome Research Institute, the National Institutes of Health Chemical Genomics Center, and the Food and Drug Administration that was established to leverage resources to advance the recommendations in the 2007 National Research Council report *Toxicity Testing in the 21st Century: A Vision and a Strategy*.

methods for understanding the principles that drive the dynamic behavior of materials, identification of a minimum set of testing platforms for comparative ENM bioactivity assessments, development and distribution of standard materials for calibrating assays, identification of more diverse sets of materials for comparative testing, more aggressive data-sharing strategies, and implementation of an informatics platform for data-mining.

Mark Wiesner, of Duke University and a member of the committee, discussed work of the Center for the Environmental Implications of Nanotechnology (funded by EPA and NSF) and the need to elucidate principles that determine environmental behavior of nanomaterials and to translate data on the environmental behavior of ENMs into risk. Dr. Wiesner asked, What nanomaterial properties and environmental conditions control the spatial and temporal distributions of nanomaterials in the environment? He emphasized the need to look at next-generation nanotechnologies, in that much of the EHS community is still focused on first-generation materials.

Development of Tools

Speakers talked about progress and innovations in the development of tools—standard test and reference materials, methods to measure ENMs in complex media, exposure and effects models, and informatics—to address the research priorities. Vincent Hackley, of the National Institute of Standards and Technology, described progress in detecting and measuring ENMs. He noted the challenge posed by the lack of adequate characterization of materials in the published toxicologic literature. That problem frustrates efforts to link ENM properties with biologic responses. There was discussion of how the research community can meet the needs for reference materials better in light of the fact that there is a gray area between traditional reference materials and "study" materials that are sufficiently homogeneous, widely available, and well characterized.

Jamie Lead, of the University of South Carolina, described integration of experimental data and their use in informing environmental-exposure models. Exposure, aggregation, bioavailability, and toxicity models are available. Dr. Lead commented that the models are more conceptual than quantitative and do not treat complex media and systems accurately. There is a need to obtain better data (coordinated with these models) so that values can be assigned to parameters and models can be validated.

Nathan Baker, of the Pacific Northwest National Laboratory, commented on the increasing number of informatics tools available for EHS nanotechnology research. A number of communities have been established to facilitate development and use of the tools, including the US-EU CoR for Databases/Ontology and Modeling, the National Cancer Informatics Program Nanotechnology working group, and the National Nanomanufacturing Network Nanoinformatics meetings. There are efforts to collect and archive metadata for data-mining and meta-analyses, such as the Nanomaterial Registry, the Nano-Bio Interactions

Knowledgebase, and the caNanoLab. However, data-mining is complicated by several factors, including the sparseness of datasets collected on different materials with different conditions and the lack of systematic variation in collected data. More incentives are needed for data-sharing and for integration of the various informatics tools. During the discussion, the role of journal editors in helping to tackle some of the issues was addressed. Dr. Baker commented that in the future it will be essential to provide a standard format for sharing data but that at this point it is important to engage the communities in the discussion.

Perspectives of Federal Agency Technical-Program Managers

Technical-program managers in EPA, NIEHS, NSF, and NIOSH discussed current and planned research efforts to address high-priority research needs, including how agency research projects and extramural funding efforts are being shaped by emerging data.

Dr. Bahadori described some of the current EHS nanotechnology research efforts in EPA, including projects in fundamental material characterization, fate and transport of materials, ecosystem health, and human health. Dr. Bahadori commented that the committee's first report will not have an immediate impact on inhouse research, but it does provide an opportunity to influence emerging fields of research through requests for application.

Barbara Karn, NSF, described efforts to move the EHS nanotechnology research program toward more complex generations of materials. Dr. Karn discussed program directions, including detailed material characterization; prevention of adverse effects; development of instrumentation, sensors, methods, and standards; a systems approach; and research to support sustainability. She described the partnership of NSF and the Consumer Products Safety Commission that was established in 2012 and expressed a hope that other research agreements can be established.

Sri Nadadur, NIEHS, discussed research funding, including the NIEHS Centers for Nanotechnology Health Implications Research (an interdisciplinary program that comprises five U19[2] and three cooperative centers and other grantees and is intended to learn how the "properties of ENMs influence their interactions with biologic systems and potential health risks) and the Nano Grand Opportunity Consortium (whose major goals are to develop reliable and reproducible assays, methods, and models that can be used to predict exposure and biologic response to ENMs in different systems and laboratories)" (NIEHS 2012). He also described the National Toxicology Program (NTP) EHS nano-

---

[2]U19 is part of the National Institute of Environmental Health Sciences Centers for Nanotechnology Health Implications Research. It is an interdisciplinary program that comprises five U19 and three cooperative centers and other grantees and is intended to increase understanding of how the properties of ENMs influence their interactions with biologic systems and potential health risks.

technology research efforts. Dr. Nadadur related how the Chemical Effects in Biological Systems database is being used to integrate and share EHS nanotechnology data generated by the NIEHS and NTP research programs.

Paul Schulte, NIOSH, commented that workers are the first people to be exposed to nanomaterials. He described a recently released report, *Filling the Knowledge Gaps for Safe Nanotechnology in the Workplace* (NIOSH 2012), that documents research progress. Dr. Schulte discussed how the research priorities outlined in the committee's first report align with NIOSH initiatives. For example, regarding the quantification and characterization of the origins of nanomaterial releases, Dr. Schulte commented that NIOSH is conducting field assessments for a variety of scenarios, including where materials are manufactured. Committee members discussed NIOSH's focus on more typical materials (for example, nanosilver), and Dr. Schulte said that the agency is trying to be more aggressive in investigating them.

There was some discussion regarding the generation of large quantities of data resulting from various federal research efforts and how to integrate the data. Committee members questioned whether there is a cross-agency effort to synthesize EHS nanotechnology data. Dr. Tinkle responded that there are efforts to coordinate planning but no collective effort in interpretation of data, which is left to the academic community. Another member rephrased the question in terms of the committee's desire to understand outcomes of federally funded research, and Dr. Tinkle responded that the NNI is looking at metrics for assessing funding programs but does not have the answers yet.

Perspectives of Stakeholders

In this session, representatives of academe, industry, labor, and environmental groups provided their perspectives on the extent of research progress and the effectiveness of stakeholder engagement in developing and implementing needed research. Consumers do not know which products that they use contain nanomaterials, and workers do not know that they may be exposed to nanomaterials in the workplace. Those comments were expressed by Carolyn Cairns, Consumers Union, and Anna Fendley, United Steel Workers, when addressing the needs of the stakeholders with whom they work. Ms. Cairns emphasized the need for linkages between research and policy. Similarly, Ms. Fendley discussed the need for better sharing of information with workers and the need to disseminate and apply information in research strategies among those who are potentially exposed. Robert (Skip) Rung, Oregon Nanoscience and Microtechnologies Institute (an economic-development organization), echoed the need for more attention to workers, given that they receive the greatest exposures. Mr. Rung expressed concern about continued regulatory uncertainty and stated that an option for companies would be to move their operations outside the United States. Seth Coe-Sullivan, a member of the committee and founder and chief technology officer of QD Vision, pointed out the need for an approach to determine what tools are needed to inform stakeholders better and to move development of the technologies forward. Dr. Coe-Sullivan, picking up on comments by Mr. Alwood, recognized that a case-by-case approach for regulating nanomaterials is not sustainable and that we need to look at categories. He stated that the research strategies are good enough but that implementation of the strategies is the problem.

REFERENCES

Keller, T.H., A. Pichota, and Z. Yin. 2006. A practical view of 'druggability'. Curr. Opin. Chem. Biol. 10(4):357-361.

NIEHS (National Institute of Environmental Health Sciences). 2012. Nanotechnology Consortiums [online]. Available: http://www.niehs.nih.gov/research/supported/dert/cospb/programs/nanotech/index.cfm [accessed Nov. 30, 2012].

NIOSH (National Institute for Occupational Safety and Health). 2012. Filling the Knowledge Gaps for Safe Nanotechnology in the Workplace. A Progress Report from the NIOSH Nanotechnology Research Center: 2004-2011. U.S. Department of Health and Human Services, Centers for Disease Control and Prevention, National Institute for Occupational Safety and Health [online]. Available: http://www.cdc.gov/niosh/docs/2013-101/pdfs/2013-101.pdf [accessed Nov. 28, 2012].

NRC (National Research Council). 2012. A Research Strategy for Environmental, Health, and Safety Aspects of Engineered Nanomaterials. Washington, DC: National Academies Press.

PCAST (President's Council of Advisors on Science and Technology). 2012. Report to the President and Congress on the Fourth Assessment of the National Nanotechnology Initiative. April 2012 [online]. Available: http://nano.gov/sites/default/files/pub_resource/pcast_2012_nanotechnology_final.pdf [accessed Apr. 18, 2013].

Reynolds, C.W. 2012. Letter to Frederick National Laboratory Staff, from Craig W. Reynolds, NCI Associate Director, Frederick National Laboratory for Cancer Research [online]. Available: http://ncifrederick.cancer.gov/News/Spotlight/FrederickNationalLab.aspx [accessed Nov. 27, 2012].